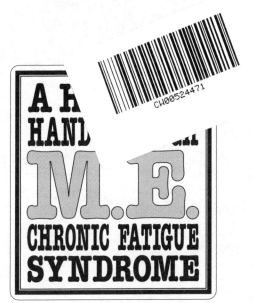

A H
HAND
M.E.
CHRONIC FATIGUE
SYNDROME

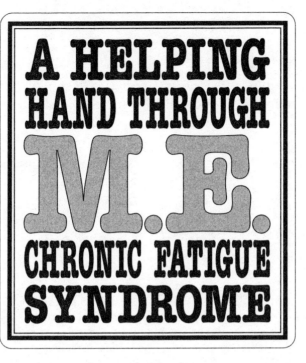

A HELPING HAND THROUGH M.E. CHRONIC FATIGUE SYNDROME

A self-help guide for sufferers and their FAMILIES

JANET HURRELL

foulsham

LONDON • NEW YORK •TORONTO • SYDNEY

foulsham

The Publishing House, Bennetts Close,
Cippenham, Slough, Berkshire, SL1 5AP

ISBN 0-572-02438-X

Copyright © 1998 Janet Hurrell

Printed by Cox & Wyman Ltd, Reading, Berks.

Contents

*This book is dedicated to
Mr Roger Rose*

Acknowledgements

I would like to thank the following people for their help and support:

My family, for putting up with a less than normal Mum for so long. My husband in particular has discovered just how much shopping I used to do – thanks Peter! – and my son Craig deserves a big hug for printing up my manuscript more than once and then altering it hundreds of times without complaint when he was already busy with his university work. I must also mention my son John for his continual prayers which I know have played their part.

My many friends who have accepted me as I am and offered help in emergencies.

Susan at Harmony Health Food Shop, Tring, who has followed the progress of my book with interest over the years.

My therapists, many of whom have become friends. I shall always be grateful for the caring help I have received, without which I would never have improved this much.

Foreword

I first met Janet Hurrell seven years ago, when as an aromatherapist I was just beginning to get a trickle of clients with M.E. and therefore had an interest in the condition. Janet at first became a client and then also a friend.

For eight years, Janet, although extremely unwell for most of the time, had been accumulating a great deal of information about M.E. She had already helped many local people with M.E. with her knowledge and her interest in their well-being, so the next obvious step was to put it all together into the form of a book to reach and help an even wider audience of sufferers. So here it is!

In March 1996, Janet started up an M.E. support group, which she still runs, in Tring. Throughout the last three years of her illness she has combined running a busy household, organising her support group and raising money for fellow M.E. sufferers. And now there is this book.

Nobody about to read this book should be under any illusions: Janet wrote this book despite her illness as well as because of it, and it has been a true labour of love. It was written with sheer determination, following the maxim that even if you can do only a very little at a time eventually the job will be completed. Janet calls this 'nibbling the elephant'. This characteristic attitude made a very big impression on me and now the word 'procrastination' has all but disappeared completely from my vocabulary.

As an holistic therapist I meet people from all walks of life but I have never met anyone like Janet Hurrell. Her sense of humour, courage, kindness and generosity are without equal and I am proud to be numbered among her friends.

Jean Caisley
M.I.F.R I.T.E.C. I.P.T.I.

September 1997

Introduction

M.E. is a strange but not new illness: it has been recognised by doctors for many years. I used to think of it as being something which had taken control of me completely, probably for ever. I now regard it simply as an illness – a complex one, certainly, but an illness which, given the right attention, can be managed and improved.

There is no quick fix for the severe problems which M.E. brings. There is no magic prescription for the illness and research into finding a cure is slow. However, there are different ways of approaching the illness:

- You can do nothing and wait until you wake up better one morning. This could take for ever.

- You can rely on whatever treatment and drugs you are offered and hope that they do the trick without causing too many side effects.

- You can learn to manage your illness, choose the remedies which suit you and look after yourself so well that your body starts to heal itself.

This book is intended to help you follow the last course, which I believe is the best choice for your route to recovery.

When I first became ill with M.E. over 10 years ago,

I knew almost nothing about it. Since then, I have read scores of books, journals and health magazine articles and asked hundreds of questions about M.E. I have experienced many different kinds of treatment and therapy, both conventional and alternative. I have learned a great deal but the 10 years have been long and slow; I now know that what I needed from the beginning was practical help and tried and tested advice from other M.E. sufferers. How much more quickly might I have recovered if I had been better informed at the outset?

A couple of years ago, a friend of mine said 'You know a lot about M.E., why don't you write a book?'. I thought this was very funny and replied that there were loads of good books on the market, written by well-qualified experts. Then I started thinking about how long it had taken me to assemble all the practical knowledge I have now and how I wished I had had it from the start. It occurred to me that I might have been completely well by now if only I had known at the outset what I have learned since. Early diagnosis would have made a big difference, too. With M.E., it is so easy to do all the wrong things if you don't know what can make you better or worse. You may even prolong the illness. So I decided to write this book, a simple, down-to-earth guide for M.E. sufferers, based on my own personal experience and feelings.

I have tried to summarise the most important information in a way which won't demand a degree in medicine to understand it. I have tried not to be too technical and I have written in small sections which you will find easier to take in. Don't try to digest it all at once, however: remember, M.E. is a very complex illness.

I have tried to be objective and even included a few topics which I personally wouldn't touch with a barge pole; but you will notice obvious leanings towards alternative medicine and natural healing methods which I have personally found to be most effective for me.

Practical information can help anyone; I truly believe that knowledge is essential for healing. In writing this book, I hope to give other sufferers of M.E. the benefit of the best of my knowledge and experience and, because my experience is limited, I have included a list of useful books which offer more detailed information.

I am not a medical expert and I am in no position to prescribe what anyone should do or not do; I cannot even say what I think you might take a crack at. I have simply put together everything I know so that fellow sufferers may find those treatments which suit them best: I hope that my book will come in handy in making you aware of what is available so that you can follow your own path with the help of advice from professional therapists. In particular, specialist advice should ALWAYS be sought for children and pregnant women.

However, the road to recovery requires more than finding the right treatment. You have to come to terms with and manage both your condition and the feelings of loneliness and utter despair it brings. So my second aim was to help other sufferers to learn to master their illness as I did and prevent it from taking charge of their lives.

If you have M.E., or are caring for someone with M.E., I hope that this book will provide you with the information and encouragement you need to find your own individual route to recovery. Don't ever give up – progress will be slow, even invisible, but if you feel just a little better on just one day, then in theory you can feel a little better every day. And each little bit will take you closer to regaining your previous good health.

Good luck to you all.

CHAPTER 1

M.E. – The Illness

What is M.E.?

M.E. stands for Myalgic Encephalomyelitis. It is a condition, not an infection. In fact, it is a number of conditions with overlapping symptoms, which will not be identical in every sufferer. The myalgic bit refers to the aching muscles, while the encephalomyelitis refers to symptoms caused by disturbance to the brain and central nervous system.

M.E. often starts after a persistent viral infection, which your immune system cannot deal with. It is as though the immune system has become unbalanced, half of it working overtime and the other half watching. The infection may be something serious, very often glandular fever, or quite trivial, but afterwards you get worse and worse instead of better.

M.E. affects the whole body and gives rise to an enormous number of symptoms, making it very difficult to identify. It is an illness of relapses and remissions and there is no one single diagnostic test for it, although doctors are working on a possible blood test to diagnose it, which is good news. Diagnosis has to be based on close examination of the symptoms and careful elimination of the possibilities of other diseases. It can, however, take time for some symptoms to develop and for the illness to 'bottom out', making the diagnostic process even more difficult.

The illness is probably as old as the hills, but has only recently received proper recognition. There are no reliable statistics relating to the number of current sufferers, as it is so hard to diagnose, but it is known that women are three times more likely to suffer than men. There may be a psychological or genetic predisposition involved in M.E., and often more than one member of a family will suffer from it.

Over the years, it has been referred to by many names, including epidemic neuromyasthenia, Royal Free disease, post-viral fatigue syndrome and chronic fatigue syndrome. The last two are the most commonly used, and certainly give some clues to the nature of the condition, but they are not strictly accurate. M.E. sufferers certainly have chronic fatigue, but not all chronic fatigue sufferers have M.E. Equally, as I have already said, many people develop M.E. after suffering a viral attack, but not everyone does.

What causes M.E.?

The causes of M.E. are, in fact, still something of a mystery. It is, however, generally accepted that some sort of stress is the primary factor, whether it be from an illness, an accident or injury (frequently to the back), overwork, hormonal imbalance or even perhaps a vaccination. One of the most common factors seems to be a recent viral infection, which may be serious – like glandular fever – or relatively mild. Even the fittest amongst us can be struck down; most of us know of an apparently healthy teenager who has suddenly been afflicted and it is not unknown amongst athletes. My own feeling is that the cause is multifaceted – there is more than one stress involved and the last problem or trauma is just the last straw.

M.E. comes in various strengths. It can start quite suddenly or creep up unnoticed over a period of months. Some people come abruptly to a halt and can do virtually nothing, while others struggle on with their lives, feeling dreadful and not knowing why, until finally it gets the better of them.

What are the symptoms of M.E.?

As we've seen, the term M.E. refers to an illness which affects not only the physical body, but also the brain and nervous system. The more I read about M.E., the more it seems to me that the brain is the crux of the problem. It is our computer and sends out constant messages to all parts of the body, but the trouble is that the messages are wrong. This is a physical problem and, so far, drugs to try and help correct some of these messages have not worked well, but doctors will keep on trying! The brains of M.E. sufferers have been found to bear strange spots, scars and lesions, although as yet no signs of inflammation, which was suspected, have been discovered. My head pain was horrific and so I still need convincing on this point, but these lesions are capable of healing themselves and, when they do, you will feel much better.

Apart from the headaches, the best-known feature

17

of M.E. is the overwhelming feeling of lethargy, unrelieved by rest or sleep and made worse by even small amounts of activity. To say you are tired is a gross understatement, as the levels of lethargy and exhaustion you experience were quite unimaginable until now.

Unfortunately, this is not only one of the major symptoms of M.E., it is also probably the most difficult to get rid of. You feel completely exhausted, unable to undertake even the smallest task. Your legs are like jelly, heavy as lead, and you are so dizzy you might as well be drunk. Your head is stuffed with cotton wool soaked in anaesthetic. If you struggle to your feet to clean your teeth, your toothbrush weighs a ton.

Your brain may also feel tired and confused; you may suffer from lack of concentration and poor memory and have difficulty forming coherent sentences. Mood swings and depression are common.

Despite the tiredness, your sleep patterns may be disturbed. You may have difficulty getting to sleep or staying asleep; you may suffer from early waking or find that you are awake all night and sleeping through the day. Vivid dreams and nightmares are also common.

You may suffer from an alarming list of symptoms: most sufferers have a sore throat and swollen glands, but not all. Most sufferers have severe joint and muscle pain, but again not all. Headaches and head pain are common, as is neck pain. You may have trouble with your digestive system. You may find

18

that you develop allergies, tinnitus, sensitivity to noise and light, urticaria, cystitis and other bladder and bowel problems.

Of course, you will not suffer from all of these and, in reality, they are not all symptoms exclusive to M.E. You may find that you have just a few or that different symptoms seem to come and go, changing all the time. The illness seems to vary from one person to another, which is what makes it so difficult to recognise and treat.

As you can see, this is not a pretty picture and needs careful handling and prompt action. As soon as you are able, try to keep a diary of your symptoms, how you feel, sleep, etc., as this will help you when you talk to your doctor. Also a record of everything you eat would be useful, as you may discover you are allergic to, or cannot tolerate, some foods.

I think of an M.E. sufferer's body as a little chemical laboratory in which all the experiments are going wrong. It takes time and effort to sort this mess out. In order to help yourself, you will have to start putting together a plan of action to strengthen your system to try and eventually heal yourself. In this book, I will help you to draw on every resource you can find to make your own plan towards recovery.

This will probably be slow and the path towards improvement never runs smoothly. It is usually two steps forward and one step back, even when things are going reasonably well. Even after a few days' or weeks' improvement, something unexpected can happen to cause a relapse. This is normal, so don't be too disappointed, and try to learn from it if possible.

In the earlier stages of M.E. there often seems to be no rhyme nor reason for what happens next but, as the illness progresses, you may feel you are just a little bit more in charge.

Diagnosis

As I have already said, there is, as yet, no definitive diagnostic test for M.E., although teams of doctors everywhere are searching for one. So unless doctors are very familiar with the symptoms of M.E., they find it difficult to diagnose. They understand the individual symptoms, like the dizziness, joint pain and gastric trouble, but do not recognise this strange combination of endless symptoms and may start by treating the worst problems individually instead of immediately regarding the illness as a whole. Your doctor will almost certainly take a blood sample, but this will not prove you have M.E. – it will only give some clues and help confirm suspicions.

To make matters even more difficult, M.E. may take some time to develop fully, so all the symptoms are not evident at the start. Also, unfortunately, M.E. is often confused with other illnesses, such as gastric, joint and psychiatric disorders. Probably the most similar conditions are chronic fatigue syndrome and severe candidiasis (see pages 75–80). The fatigue of multiple sclerosis is said to be indistinguishable from M.E. at the outset: the symptoms of fibromyalgia can be incredibly like M.E. and some doctors even think it is a non-paralytic form of polio. As M.E. frequently follows a viral illness like flu, it is often assumed to be post-viral debility, which is nasty, but just not the same.

To help you and your doctor tackle the problem, let's have a look at the most prominent features by which M.E. can be recognised:

1. The main distinguishing marker, as I have already mentioned, is the lethargy which is unrelieved by sleep and made worse by even small amounts of activity. There is nearly always a time lag between the activity and the exhaustion, which is out of all proportion to the task undertaken.

2. Sleep patterns are disturbed. There is difficulty in getting to sleep, or staying asleep; early wakening is common and often the sufferer will be asleep all day and awake all night. You may have vivid dreams and nightmares.

3. M.E. sufferers have trouble with their brains; poor memory, lack of concentration, trouble finding words and so on. They also feel dizzy and unco-ordinated. Mood swings and bouts of depression are common.

4. Most (but not all) sufferers have a sore throat and swollen glands.

5. Most (but not all) sufferers have joint and muscle pain. Head and neck pain is common.

6. Gastric and bowel problems are widespread among the majority.

7. There is an enormous variety of symptoms, which may last or may disappear temporarily, only to return when you least expect them.

I had candida and allergies and was very sensitive to noise. Some sufferers may also have more serious conditions of the heart, liver and thyroid. I will deal with the full list of symptoms in a later chapter, but for now we shall content ourselves with the main ones which help towards diagnosis.

Both Action for M.E. and the M.E. Association (see page 179) produce good material to help you and your doctor with diagnosis. The factsheets available from Action for M.E. are particularly helpful and they also run a 24-hour telephone helpline which gives information on causes and symptoms of M.E. (see page 175).

Is it catching?

There is no such thing as an M.E. virus or bacterium, so it can't be passed from person to person. However, if two predisposed people are together and in contact with the same trigger factor, for example, glandular fever, they would probably (although not certainly) both get it, but not from each other. This may explain why there is a high incidence of M.E. amongst teachers and nurses.

Am I going bonkers?

Definitely not! But you should realise that M.E. is a serious illness which affects the whole body, including your brain. The poor brain gets a real bashing in M.E. Your memory will not function quickly, your reactions will be sluggish and your attention span will be short. An illness which has such devastating and weakening effects will inevitably affect your state of mind too, and the severity of this prolonged illness will often produce bouts of depression. However this does NOT mean that you are somehow unbalanced in any way, and you should never allow anyone to suggest (as may well happen) that the whole thing is all in your mind. Our brain problems are physical, not mental, ones.

However, if you suffer from prolonged depression, you may need to seek expert help. There are herbal remedies which may relieve the misery – KIRA tablets, which contain hypericum, are found to help some people, and I would recommend Bach Flower Rescue Remedy.

Anyone with M.E. may find cognitive behavioural therapy (see page 86) helpful to them, as would sufferers of many other severe illnesses. This is a very effective, direct form of counselling and is available on the NHS.

In the past doctors have very readily prescribed Prozac (see page 88) to M.E. sufferers. However, it is now accepted that this does not help everyone and in some cases may make the sufferer feel worse.

Learning to cope

This is a great big problem, but cope we must. The first step is to accept what has happened. If you react

23

by battling inside yourself, saying 'It's not fair!' or 'I will not accept this, I am going to ignore it until it goes away', you will get nowhere. Once you quieten down, relax and start planning the future, you are taking the first step towards improving.

Keeping a positive mental attitude definitely kept me going. I tried to think of all the different things I could try in order to get better and made sure I always had another card up my sleeve, so that if one thing didn't work I would try something else. I now realise that it is not enough simply to take one or two measures and expect to get well; we have to persevere with the whole package and that does take some dedication.

I have also consoled myself with the fact that I did stand a chance of recovering and at least I could be ill in comfort, which is more than can be said for some people. I have kept telling myself that everyone has a really bad patch at some time in their life and this has been mine. When it is all over, I shall appreciate life more fully.

Health is a combination of mental, physical and emotional factors. Your immune system is strongly influenced by the mind as well as what is physically happening to your body. It is fair to say that your mental attitude is a powerful part of your recovery system. A positive attitude can really help, but don't think of it as a magic wand. M.E. is a complex illness and takes a lot of sorting out. Nevertheless, if you can maintain a good positive attitude most of the time, you are much more likely to return to good health all the sooner.

Aiming for recovery

The other factor which is vital to your recovery is your mental strength. As I have said, you have, first of all, to accept the fact that you are ill but you also have to learn a whole new lifestyle to cope with your illness. The battle against M.E. is a strategic one as much as a physical one. You will have to learn to recognise your enemy and formulate a plan of action to deal with it. You will find that it is a long, slow process, with one step back for every two forward, at the beginning, at least. You will have to come to terms with relapses, disappointments, setbacks and sheer frustration. You will have to find strength inside yourself for all this.

If you have a faith, this will undoubtedly be a source of great comfort to you. I consider myself a Christian, although not too hot on the technical side, and I did quite a lot of praying. I think that everyone with M.E. probably does, even if it is for the first time in their life. There is nothing wrong with a daily prayer for the strength to cope. You may also receive help in getting better and even the ability to learn some of life's lessons from it all. I certainly feel that I have had so much help from Upstairs, that I feel more in touch than ever with my God and confident that I am going in the right direction. However you do it, muster all your resources in your fight towards recovery.

Will I ever really recover?

Current statistics say that 20 per cent sufferers of M.E. make a complete recovery; this may seem like a rather small proportion but I am talking about COMPLETE recovery. Of the remainder, the vast majority reach a point where they can live more or less normal lives, with care. Only a small percentage remain very ill for good, or improve at first, only to relapse into a chronic condition.

I am not a great one for statistics, however, and I most certainly don't think you should believe everything you read. Much that has been printed in the press is inaccurate, incomplete and misleading and, if I had believed everything I read, I would certainly be worse now instead of steadily improving. Of course, you should read up as much as you can – the more knowledge you have, the better you can manage your illness – but get as much information as you can from reputable sources, such as the M.E. Association (see page 179). What is really important is that you seek an early diagnosis to give yourself the best chance of recovery.

Research into M.E.

There is an increasing amount of research on M.E. going on at the moment in Britain, where the main stalwart is Professor Behan at Glasgow University who, with a team of 20 scientists, has been studying M.E. since the 1970s. There is further research going on in Europe, a great deal in America and a perhaps surprising interest in New Zealand where they have suffered large outbreaks.

The Glasgow team has discovered the effectiveness of Efamol Marine, a natural product made up of 80 per cent primrose oil and 20 per cent marine fish oil.

In Southampton, a team of scientists have been working on magnesium injections which appear to help some sufferers (see pages 89–91).

American research has produced two drugs with anti-viral qualities, which have shown some success. However, neither of these is currently available in Britain, and one, Ampligen, has been put on hold while further investigations on possible side effects are carried out. The other, Kutapressin, is still in its infancy, and also needs published trials before it can be marketed. Unfortunately, to date, the British government has funded next to no research at all.

CHAPTER 2

Common Symptoms and How to Handle Them

In Chapter 1, I gave a depressingly long list of the symptoms and conditions associated with M.E. Now we shall look at how we can best control the commonest of these symptoms in order to make life more bearable for the M.E. patient.

Fatigue

Fatigue, along with pain, is probably the very worst feature of M.E. At the onset of the illness, I used to think that I could cope with being tired if only the pain would subside. When it eventually did, I discovered that the fatigue could actually be the most severe, restricting and seemingly everlasting symptom of all.

When you are first ill, it is important that you have plenty of rest: this helps the chances of complete recovery and lessens the possibility of the illness becoming chronic. As you improve, it is essential that you manage your activity carefully, using your limited energy in little 'bites'. It is tempting to keep going too long to finish off a job, but if this puts you to bed, you will soon realise that you will actually get more done by stopping and starting, than by being laid up and having to stop completely! As a rule we should only use up 70 per cent of our energy before stopping. This is difficult to calculate, especially if we actually feel quite good. Only experience will tell you when to stop and, while you are learning, err on the safe side: stop *before* you are tired, not *when* you are tired.

When you are too poorly to do anything much but lie down, remember that mental activity will tire you too. The most restful activity is listening quietly to music or tapes. You don't have to concentrate for this. I don't know what I would have done without the television for company, but even this will tire you as it takes concentration and it is probably not advisable to watch it all day long. It also hurts the eyes in long sessions. Remember that while you used to watch TV, talk, knit or read all at the same time, this will be too much now and it is enough to cope with one thing at a time.

Relapses may be caused by physical, mental or emotional stress; infections and viruses; injections, vaccinations, antibiotics and anaesthetics, and possibly other drugs too. Even being too hot or cold will upset you.

Dizziness

Dizziness and 'spaced out' feelings are common in M.E. sufferers and may be caused by high or low blood pressure.

Many sufferers feel dizzy on rising as the blood

pressure temporarily plummets. When I had bad patches like this, I moved more slowly. Taking a little quality salt may also be useful for low blood pressure dizziness, but it won't cure the problem completely. Be careful not to overdo it and do consult your doctor.

Solgar's Hawthorn Berry herbal tablets and sublingual vitamin B_{12} may help and gingko bilboba is also recommended to help circulation as long as you don't have heart problems.

When doing yoga recently, I realised that one position with the legs in the air would probably help bring the blood back towards the heart. Some people recommend lying on the floor with your legs up against the wall.

Other causes of dizziness are hyperventilation (see pages 35–6), low blood sugar (see pages 36–7) and vitamin B_{12} deficiency. It may also be associated with candida and mercury toxicity.

Pain

Apart from fatigue, pain is the real bugbear of M.E. sufferers. All sorts of pain: severe, splitting headaches; stabbing pains in temples and ears; pains in your calves, shins and thighs; knee pains that will literally stop you in your tracks; twitching, aching muscles; pains in your neck and shoulders; chest pains, usually brought on by activity – the list really seems endless.

With the pain comes a host of things to drag you

down: tiredness, stiffness, sleep disturbance, poor memory and concentration, depression and mood swings; it all adds up to real misery. So what can you do to help yourself?

Doctors can prescribe pain-killing drugs and you can buy effective analgesics over the counter of any chemist. But you may find that these do not help or, worse, that they produce side effects. The long-term use of painkillers can cause stomach bleeding, digestive problems, dizziness, fluid retention and even headaches! Natural herbal remedies for pain relief, such as white willow bark and feverfew, are much kinder and just as effective.

Good results may be obtained from physiotherapy (see pages 108–10), acupuncture (see pages 93–5), homeopathy (see pages 99–101), reflexology (see pages 110–11) and, in some cases, massage (see pages 104–7). Magnetic therapy (see pages 101–3) is worth trying too. However, don't try massage if you suffer from back problems or oedema in that area as it may make things worse (see page 106).

At one point I had a recurring bad pain in my neck and shoulders and could hardly move at all. My physiotherapist/acupuncturist treated it with electrical pads and acupuncture and it disappeared very quickly. This made me realise that neck pain, at least, does not have to be a long-lasting M.E. problem. Anyone can have it but equally anyone can get rid of it.

Better, perhaps, are gentle stretching exercises or Tai Chi. I have recently had great success with yoga, but couldn't do it at first as it is far more strenuous than it looks. You can get information about specially designed courses of gentle remedial yoga from the M.E. Association (see page 179).

M.E. legs

With the pain, you may also suffer from 'M.E. legs'. They feel so heavy, yet weak as jelly; they don't want to walk. Knees can be a particularly bad problem. Sometimes you will be too ill to walk at all and if your legs are painful, this is a signal to rest.

Many people have symptoms of strong, sore pains in their calves. This can also occur in other areas of the legs. I have experienced pain of this sort in the front upper leg muscles and also had tender swelling and pain up the shins. Apparently, lactic acid is the culprit. It is the natural waste product from exercise, or in our case, just pottering! Unfortunately we are using up our limited energy faster than healthy people and getting rid of it very, very slowly. It is the build-up that causes the pain.

Rest helps but you should also try rubbing your muscles several times a day to disperse the lactic acid. This can be done in bed, on the sofa or in the bath. Remember, however, getting rid of the pain is a relief but it doesn't mean that you have recharged your energy. Take care!

My massage therapist friend tells me that the toxins are best eliminated by rubbing the leg upwards from ankle to knee and, if necessary, from knee to thigh.

Fibromyalgia

If you have a lot of pain in your shoulders or down your back, you may have fibromyalgia, or fibrositis, as it used to be called. The symptoms are tender spots in the muscles and muscles which feel like stiff cords, even when relaxed. I found that Guaiacum, a homoeopathic remedy, was particularly effective in relieving this pain. Guaiacum is noted for its ability to help joint pain, loss of flexibility, catarrh and sore throats. The theory is that the guai in the remedy melts away the build-up of phosphates in our joints and muscles, literally 'freeing us up'. Incidentally, people with a lot of tartar on their teeth may notice that this is also reduced. My teeth now need much less frequent attention from the hygienist and my shoulders are far looser.

Other good herbal remedies for natural pain relief are white willow bark and feverfew, which is recommended for migraine sufferers. Sometimes simple relaxation, warmth or a bag of frozen peas placed on the affected area may provide the answer.

Gentle exercises can be very relaxing and may also help to ward off pain and stiffness. Try the following, but stop immediately if you feel any additional discomfort:

1. Gently nod your head, at least ten times. It has to be a very shallow movement, like one of those nodding dogs in the back of a car. The chin will only go up and down about 2.5 cm (1 inch). Repeat this exercise about ten times a day. You should not expect miracles, but if you stick at it you could feel

a lot better in a day or two. Even if you are seriously ill, you will find you can nod whilst lying down. I have found that it is best to keep up the exercise for a few days after the pain has gone, as it tends to come back.

2. Extend your chin forwards, then back, rather like a chicken. Again, it is a very slight movement.

3. Shrug your shoulders up and down.

4. Brace your shoulders back, and, with slightly bent arms, stick your chest out, then relax.

Hyperventilation

This is sometimes called over-breathing. People who hyperventilate are breathing too fast in the upper chest near the neck, when they should be breathing quite slowly low down in the diaphragm area. Many people with M.E. could be hyperventilating without realising it. If it is a mild problem, it is difficult to recognise. If it is a very severe problem, you may need expert help, particularly if you are prone to panic attacks.

Hyperventilation causes an imbalance of oxygen and carbon dioxide in the body and this may lead to symptoms like pins and needles, muscle weakness, noise sensitivity, dizziness, sweating, anxiety and even nightmares. Ideally, you should go to a physiotherapist and learn relaxation and proper breathing techniques.

However, if you are prone to hyperventilation, you

can learn to control it yourself. Keep checking your breathing by putting one hand on your middle at the lower end of your ribs and try to breathe slowly, feeling the air going in and out at that area. Check with the other hand on the upper chest near the neck that this area is hardly moving. It takes quite a long time for this to become a habit but, if you know you have a problem and constantly check yourself, you will improve.

Relaxation tapes are also a very good way to unwind, as is listening to very relaxing music quietly. The more relaxed you are, the easier it will be to breathe in a slow, relaxed way. I used a little reminder phrase to help me remember to breathe correctly – 'low and slow'.

Hypoglycaemia (low blood sugar)

Many sufferers have trouble keeping their blood sugar levels stable, which can leave them feeling even more dizzy, weak and shaky (as if they weren't already!). Some possible causes of hypoglycaemia could be: sugary diet, getting too hungry, stress, food allergy, vitamin deficiency and even tea, coffee and alcohol.

Some people mistakenly think that cramming down a Mars Bar will sort the problem out. Delicious though it is, sugary food is the worst possible thing you can take for hypoglycaemia. It may give you a quick whiz of energy for a short while, but it will be followed by an even dizzier and hungrier patch later on as your sugar levels fly up and down.

36

Frequent small snacks and small meals will help to keep your sugar levels stable. Aim for lots of good quality protein, nuts and seeds, vegetables, fruit and foods high in fibre, such as wholegrains, peas and beans. Sometimes it is difficult to know what to eat between meals. If your diet permits, an oat biscuit or a Ryvita, an apple, a banana, or some nuts or seeds might help. If, like me, you have a high allergy load, you might find yourself raiding the fridge for a couple of spoons of hummus, some home-made pâté or soup. I have even had a quarter of cockles or a fried egg! This may sound strange for elevenses, but it is a lot healthier than reaching for a sugary biscuit and a cup of coffee.

Little and often is a satisfactory way of eating. Small meals are more digestible too, and well suited to someone with a poor appetite or digestive troubles. Some nutritionists recommend protein for breakfast to 'stoke up the boiler'. Starchy breakfasts make some people sleepy and may be less satisfying. With a little trial and error, you will discover which is best for you, depending on your lifestyle, appetite and digestive system.

Never go to bed hungry!

If you are really concerned about your condition, it would be advisable to have a test for diabetes with your doctor.

Plumbing problems

M.E. sufferers often have plumbing problems. Sufferers often cannot hold their water normally and need to pay frequent visits to the lavatory. Sometimes there may be mild to acute discomfort, which leads to cystitis. There are several preparations available from the chemist which are good for this condition and I found herbal Antitis from health shops to be very effective (and also a lot cheaper).

However, it is no good living on pills if you don't know the cause behind cystitis. Unless there is a genuine infection which does not respond to any treatment, antibiotics will only make matters worse, causing a vicious cycle of returning problems.

Food allergy can play havoc with your bladder and after you discover which foods and drinks upset you, you will feel a lot more comfortable. Too much acidic food can make matters worse, e.g. tomatoes, plums and even bought fresh fruit juices, due to their hidden additives and invisible yeastiness.

Careful eating and drinking and lots of water can make a big difference. Cranberry juice is often recommended for cystitis. However, it always contains sugar and will also be 'yeasty' and therefore not always suitable. Solgar have a cranberry pill which may help.

Irritable bowel syndrome (IBS)

Most M.E. sufferers have some kind of trouble with their digestive system. It is often very bad at the onset of the illness but can continue to be a nuisance indefinitely. Symptoms may include wind, bloating, gripy pains, belching, diarrhoea or constipation, or both alternating. The condition could be made worse by poor diet, lack of fibre, food allergy, anxiety, drugs, smoking, stress and depression.

So what can you do to help? Listening to relaxing tapes may help with stress. Eating more fibre or taking psyllium husks could help to keep you regular and give your inside a bit of a spring clean. BioCare's Colon Care capsules contain cascara, golden seal, pepsin and psyllium, and you may find these helpful. In spite of some strange things that are said about it, the Hay Diet (see pages 119–20) can help a lot too. There are various herbal preparations which could help and herbalists often recommend slippery elm. Peppermint oil may be another useful option.

I have read extensively about the digestive system and confess to finding it a complicated subject. However, one message comes across loud and clear: there is a close connection between the health and condition of the colon and the general health of the individual, so look after your insides in the best way you possibly can! Eat a healthy, balanced diet with plenty of fibre and if you must use a laxative, try a gentle, herbal one.

For quite a while, everyone turned to wheat bran to solve their problems. This is now thought to be too harsh and abrasive and could even make matters worse. Oat bran is more gentle (and gluten-free) and a diet with sufficient fibre is recommended, augmented with psyllium husks and linseeds. I find psyllium husks are very good but some people are sensitive to them.

39

It has been suggested to me by one knowledgeable gentleman that a sluggish system in M.E. sufferers is probably due to the fact that their muscles don't have the physical power to push the food from top to bottom efficiently.

Sleeping problems

Sleep should be a dream word. It takes us away from aching reality with hopes of a better tomorrow. But is it? M.E. sufferers need an enormous amount of sleep and rest and are usually able to sleep well when first ill. As the illness progresses, however, it is very common for sleep patterns to become disturbed. Getting to sleep can be difficult and staying asleep even worse! There are so many things that can wake us up – nightmares, frequent trips to the loo, pain, hunger, tinnitus and palpitations. My biggest problem was an over-active brain and there were some nights when nothing seemed to help. However, relaxation and breathing techniques did sometimes help and are worth learning.

Herbal and homoeopathic remedies available from health food shops may help some people. It will involve trial and error, but it's worth it if you can find something helpful. I found herbal remedies bought over the counter were ineffective, but I am now sleeping well as a result of homoeopathic treatment prescribed by an expert. This is the first good sleep I have had for ages.

Different pills suit different problems. Arnica is said to be helpful for poor sleep, but try coffea if you have a busy, restless mind. The Bach Flower

Remedy, olive, is said to alleviate exhaustion without sleep, and white chestnut is recommended for a restless brain. Homoeopathy is *not* a DIY therapy, however, and it is not wise to go on dosing yourself indefinitely on herbal remedies without understanding or supervision.

Boots sell a wrist band which can be used on the acupuncture sleep point but I found the acupuncture needle more effective. Sometimes, taking calcium at night may help. Obviously, it is wise to avoid caffeine near bedtime, in drinks such as tea, coffee, chocolate and cola.

One of the most common sleep disturbances is early waking. Even if it is easy to get to sleep (which isn't always the case), it is a very usual pattern to wake in the early hours and not be able to resettle. This does get very wearing night after night but don't let it actually worry you. Just rest the best you can and sleep during the day if you need to. This sleep pattern is called sleep reversal. It doesn't last for ever, and is not a cause for concern.

If you sleep a lot during the day your family may worry that you will not sleep at night. It simply does not work like that with M.E. You need all the sleep or rest you can get, day or night, or both! If you try to be more active during the day, thinking you will be more tired and so sleep better, forget it! You could finish up more ill and sleeping less. If you resist sleep or rest during the day in the hope of a better night, this doesn't work either. Being overtired can make sleep very difficult and your health will deteriorate further.

However much sleep you get at first, if you have M.E. you will still wake unrefreshed, but in the long-term, only sleep can help a very overtired body.

If you decide to take sleeping pills, make sure you know exactly what is involved. They may or may not work; they give a poor quality of sleep; they give side effects (like more M.E.); you may discover you need larger and larger doses for the same effect; you may quickly become dependent and find it difficult to stop. They should only be taken as an emergency measure occasionally or for just a week or so, to re-establish your sleeping pattern. They should not be regarded as a long-term solution, especially as drugs may suppress the immune system, the very thing we are trying to improve.

There are a few precautions you can take to prevent nights being even worse than they need to be. Avoid evening baths and showers, which can invigorate before you go to bed; also over-activity (the chance would be a fine thing!). Wind down and relax at bedtime, with a relaxation tape or quiet music if you find it helps you.

Just one last thing it may be helpful to know: sleep tends to get difficult after catching viruses and this may last for weeks. Eventually, as you improve and your energy starts returning again, sleep often improves slowly too.

Research has shown that the brain wave pattern in M.E. sufferers who are sleeping is the same as those in healthy people who are awake – food for thought!

Sore throat and swollen glands

I think almost all M.E. sufferers have this at first, and it often lasts for a very long time. It was 18 months before my sore throat and swollen glands started to calm down to a 'just now and then' basis! Your doctor may prescribe antibiotics if he thinks there is an infection present; if there is not, they will have no beneficial effect and should be avoided.

Sore throats are very common in people whose immune system is weak. Again, there are analgesic tablets, sprays and lozenges available over the counter but I prefer to use the herbal remedies available at your health shop. To soothe a sore throat, I would recommend Ricola blackcurrant Swiss herb lozenges which are sugar-free. They do also contain menthol, which may interfere with homoeopathic remedies, and aspartame. Sucking Solgar Flavo-zinc lozenges (one a day) may also help fight infections as will gargling with propolis tincture, which can be swallowed. It helps kill bugs and has a slightly anaesthetic effect. Even gargling with salt water may give relief.

As you improve, you will find that your glands are up one day and down the next until the problem finally disappears.

Stress

Most M.E. sufferers feel stressed or are stressed, but they are not aware of it. This is not surprising as the illness alone is enough to stress anyone. There may also be problems with sleep, money, work, family, etc. Even the weather, the temperature and noise may be stressful.

Stress can lead to unpleasant symptoms such as headaches, insomnia, high blood pressure, depression, palpitations and muscle tension. Unfortunately, our immobility hinders our ability to 'work off the adrenaline' and, as our bodies are functioning below par anyway, our handling of adrenaline is rather inadequate. I have a theory that this load of excess adrenaline we carry aggravates and overlaps with our M.E. symptoms. It is difficult to tell what is causing what any more!

So what can we do about it? Ideally, it would help to get rid of the problems causing the stress in the first place. This is not always possible and the illness is likely to last some time. However, stress can be helped by relaxation (see page 109). Also vitamins and minerals can make a difference, as can changing your diet. Stephen Terrass's book *Stress – How Your Diet Can Help* (see page 176) is most helpful in understanding this common but complicated problem.

Sweating and shivering

These are common problems; you will mostly feel cold and shivery (with cold hands and icy feet) but will very likely be sweating a lot in between times. I used to have the strangest sweating at the beginning of the illness. A hot wave would sweep over me, but my face would feel cold and just slightly clammy to the touch. I was also very pale! It is really important to have a nice warm room in the house where you will spend most of your time; being cold tenses muscles and is miserable, stressful and not conducive to healing.

If the room isn't quite warm enough, you will feel cold, but if it gets too hot and stuffy, you could find yourself sweating non-stop. You will find that you are frequently adjusting the thermostat. Try to let the room temperature and your body settle down together. When I had attacks of sweating (several times a minute), I found the only way to keep it at bay was to lower the temperature of the room slightly and wear layers of warm jumpers! Once you can recognise this problem, you will find your own best solution.

Part of our brain called the hypothalamus is at the root of the problem. It regulates our temperature and could be described as our thermostat. It seems to become very sensitive and erratic in many M.E. sufferers. It is also responsible for irregular sleeping patterns, loss of libido and appetite, lethargy, palpitations and bladder troubles. It really has a lot to answer for!

Unfortunately, nothing can stop this unpleasant sweating occurring except time and healing. However, you can avoid hot baths and too much hot sun, which will make it worse, along with too much activity that you are not ready for.

More recently I discovered another helpful tip. Just as a bath which is too hot will make me feel weak and dizzy all day, so will a humid bathroom. I find it very helpful if I can keep the steam down: I do this by running an inch or so of cold water first and then adding the hot, followed by both until the right temperature is reached. Don't stay in too long either. You may find a shower a refreshing alternative but again, don't stand in it very long; you could still get dizzy and it's further to fall.

At the other end of the scale, remember, warm clothes, cosy slippers and a hot water bottle can be a great comfort if you are too cold.

Tinnitus (noises in the ear)

I experienced this for some years before I realised it was definitely connected with my M.E., after which time I have read about it several times. In retrospect, I think it was quite possibly caused by ear wax and catarrh. Apparently, food allergies, poor circulation, coffee and smoking may also play a part.

Tinnitus is a real nuisance, especially at night when it is quiet. I found it to be much worse as the night wore on and this made it more difficult to sleep in the early hours. If it is on only one side and not too loud, muffling your ear into the pillow will help a little. I found this method a bit suffocating with two ears! When it was really bad, I tried wax earplugs in desperation. They only help if you push them well in: then they are rather uncomfortable but it may be the lesser of the two evils.

During the day, household noises, TV or quiet music help to mask the irritating humming or buzzing noise which is constantly present in your ear. If, however, it becomes a serious nuisance, you would be advised to approach a doctor about a masking device. This makes more pleasant noises in your ear to drown out the nasty ones.

You could also try playing music directly into your ear through a Walkman but do be sure to keep it very quiet as loud noise in the ears is said to be a cause of tinnitus and deafness.

I discovered that the worse I felt generally, the worse the tinnitus tended to be. Apparently, fatigue, stress and noise aggravate it, so avoiding these will help, but unfortunately there is no magic pill to cure it. As my health in general improved on a holistic homoeopathic remedy tailored especially for my needs, so my tinnitus improved. I only notice it now if I cheat on my diet!

CHAPTER 3

Starting to Help Yourself

I think this is a good time to talk about some of the psychological/emotional aspects of your illness. It is very important, if you are going to learn to cope with the physical side of M.E., that you are able to put yourself in the right frame of mind first.

From the very beginning, you will have to learn patience. Recovering from M.E. is a very long, slow business; each step on the road to recovery can take weeks, or even months. You have to learn to wait and watch and wait some more. You also have to learn to listen patiently whilst family and friends talk about their busy lives, what new jobs they are taking on, sports they are trying, holidays they are enjoying – while you can't join in. You may feel that you are living in a glass cage, that you are in prison and you don't know the date of your release. This all takes some getting used to.

You have to learn not to overstretch or overestimate yourself. You must pace yourself, and not rush yourself even when you think you are making progress. You must learn not to make promises you may not be able to keep. This is particularly hard if you have a job that you are desperate to get back to. You may feel that you are letting other people down, especially if you have been used to helping out on committees, or organising events for your church or your children's schools. Try to learn to hold back.

You will undoubtedly find that you will be given a great deal of advice, all of it well-intentioned and 'for your own good', but perhaps not well-founded and not what you want to hear. Aim at all times to manage your illness your own way, the best way for you, with information from reliable sources (like this book!) and learn to stick to your guns. Your friends and even your own family will probably find it difficult to get used to the new you – a lot of explaining will be needed, so prepare yourself to do this but only when you feel up to it.

You may find you are being talked into things you don't want to do and treatments you don't feel happy about. Your brain may be muddled and confused, so don't make any decisions until you have had time to think about them. You may even feel your doctor is not as sympathetic as you would like. If this is the case, try at first to educate him or her, but if you think you really need to change to a different doctor, Action for M.E.(see page 179) have lists of suitable doctors in your area and will advise you on how to make the necessary arrangements.

There are many areas in which you can take positive steps to aid your recovery.

Activity

After a few weeks or months of illness, you may start to feel just a little bit better and want to start doing something at last. Don't be tempted to do too much, however. It is vitally important that you pace yourself gradually, according to how you feel. The amount you can undertake will vary from day to day and has a direct relationship with your health and energy *on that particular day*. We all make mistakes at first but trial, error and experience soon give us a good idea of how much we dare attempt.

Start extremely slowly and, even when you feel considerably better, always take things a little at a time. It is much better to alternate short tasks with rests in between than to keep going all morning and rest all afternoon. Our bodies are like power stations run on batteries, but the trouble with M.E. sufferers is that our batteries go flat very quickly, much quicker than other people's. We have only limited energy available and it is very soon used up.

If we carry on with flat batteries, we get exhausted. If we are in poor health, a 10-minute task can flatten us for the rest of the day or longer. The unexpected danger occurs when we feel much better and keep going too long, then later that day, or more often during the next two days, exhaustion sets in. There is nearly always a time lag between the exertion and the exhaustion.

It would seem that it is also possible for a relapse to take place after doing just a *little bit* too much every day without realising it. This is the most difficult situation to judge as we tend to carry on if things seem to be going well. Relapses can sometimes happen for no apparent reason, which is the most disappointing of all.

When you read books and articles about M.E., you will constantly come across the phrase 'graduated exercise'. This is supposed to mean that you can gradually do a little more as you feel able. Unfortunately, this phrase can be misinterpreted as 'graduated sport'. Sport of any kind, even if you are improving, is a very dangerous undertaking. I know of sufferers now in wheelchairs who have lived to regret it. I have invented my own phrase which I feel is far more appropriate for M.E. sufferers in their early stages of recovery – 'graduated pottering'!

When you have recovered sufficiently, you may be able to do some very gentle exercises, which will tone and relax your muscles and help circulation. My physiotherapist gave me some which are little more than movements rather than actual exercises. I only do them on my good days.

Your energy is a valuable commodity to be used with great care. If you have nothing in the bank and take your credit card for a shopping spree, you are spending money you can't afford and will end up in real trouble. In the same way, if you continue to use up energy with nothing left in your batteries, you will be in worse trouble! Both will catch up with you in the end, take my word for it.

You may find that, when you get absorbed with or excited about an activity you are involved in, the excitement and adrenaline can keep you going artificially, when your real energy is, in fact, used up. It is best to learn your own limitations, get to know your own body, be very aware of what is going on and pace your day safely and accordingly. Try to use up only 70 per cent of your energy (if only we had a meter!). When you can safely manage your current workload and consistently feel about 80 per cent normal for several weeks, then you might warily try taking on a tiny bit more.

Some M.E. sufferers constantly do too much, then relapse and spend a long time resting up again, repeating this cycle. This is no way to get better. If I had to invent a slogan for M.E., it would be 'Catch up slowly'! The inability to recover normally after exertion is the main marker of M.E. Bear this in mind every day. Exertion of any kind can only be undertaken when the sufferer feels up to it, and some seriously ill people have to wait a long time before they can attempt anything. Do remember, however, that lethargy and lying in bed seem to promote further lethargy and at some point you will have to make an effort for five minutes and break the vicious circle.

Eating and drinking

It is most important that you eat a balanced, sensible diet in order to aid your recovery and then maintain good health. Full details of diets are given in a separate chapter, but there are some general guidelines which are worth including here.

Avoid stimulants, particularly caffeine, which is found in tea, coffee, chocolate (sorry!) and cola drinks. It will keep you awake at night, however tired you may be, adding further to your fatigue and sleep problems.

Alcohol is another thing to avoid at all costs. You may feel, when you are particularly low, that a drink will give you a lift. Unfortunately, very few M.E. sufferers can tolerate alcohol, even in the small quantities. If it can make a healthy person woozy, just think what it will do to someone who is already weak and wobbly. It won't help your liver either, overloaded as it is with the burden of trying to support your body's defences.

Alcoholic drinks are full of yeasts, chemicals and concentrated fruit sugars, all of which are bad for sufferers of M.E. Alcohol also depletes the body of vitamins, particularly vitamin B, zinc and magnesium, all vital to good health.

Perhaps fortunately, M.E. sufferers seem to react very badly to alcohol – I get splitting headaches and I know of one person who was physically sick if she accidentally consumed any – so you are probably unlikely to want it anyway!

One last thing to avoid in your diet, surprisingly, is sugar. Again you may find that you cannot tolerate it and feel better if you avoid it altogether. This is a good thing as it is laden with unwanted calories, promotes hypoglycaemia (see pages 36–7) and provides a banquet for candida (see page 75) to thrive on. It may also affect the ability of your white blood cells to fight infection.

Viruses

Do your very best to avoid catching viruses as these will really pull you down. Inevitably, you are almost bound to catch something from other people during the winter unless you are completely cocooned. Rest is the only answer for relapse. If you catch a mild cold, the sort you have probably had before, you may not be too badly affected, but if something a bit new and nastier comes along, it could make you quite poorly and tired for much longer.

As for medicines, I will leave these to your own judgement and that of your doctor, but do try to avoid antibiotics unless you are gravely ill, as these could do you more harm than good. I am pleased to say that, since I have been on homoeopathy (see pages 98–101), I am recovering more quickly than I used to.

If you do catch a cold, Boots sell an electrical appliance called a 'Virotherm', which is an updated and more efficient version of the old steam treatment for colds. Some M.E. patients have found it helpful in getting rid of colds and viruses more quickly, especially if they are caught early.

Stress

I have laid great emphasis on the care which has to be taken to avoid physical stress and overactivity, but it is not always appreciated that emotional and mental stress can damage your health just as much. In my opinion, they are even worse. If you are worried, stressed or emotionally upset, your health is likely to deteriorate very quickly.

We know that stress, sadness and depression are bad for the health; conversely, relaxation, happiness, and

55

laughter are good for the health. Admittedly, there is not a lot to laugh about when you have M.E., but you should try to take the time and if necessary seek help to sort out any problems that are bugging you, lest they prevent your improvement.

I realise this is very difficult for some people who can no longer work; they have financial problems, children to care for and, through no fault of their own, are throwing a lot of worry and pressure on to their families. Try to remember that worrying about problems won't make them go away and sometimes therapies like relaxation techniques or listening to soothing tapes can help you to relax, cope better or at least come to terms with the problems. I think it is essential to be able to talk to helpful, under-standing people too. This could be a friend or relative, or even a trained counsellor, as many doctors nowadays recommend counselling as part of the treatment for M.E. sufferers.

One type of stress that you may not have heard of is geopathic stress. It is believed that this is caused when the natural radiation which rises up through the earth is distorted by weak electro-magnetic fields created by water, mineral concentrations, fault lines and underground cavities. The wavelengths of the natural radiation thus become harmful to all living organisms.

If you sleep in a geopathically stressed place, the more you sleep, the worse you will feel. During sleep your brain is supposed to rest and heal your body. However, if you sleep over harmful earth rays, your brain will be constantly fighting this stress and will be unable to heal you properly, so that you will always wake up tired. Tests using an apparatus called a VEGA machine (see page 73) will confirm if you are geopathically stressed.

You can have your home checked by trained dowsers who claim they can detect geopathic stress, and a machine called a RadiTech has been produced by a company called Dulwich Health (see page 182), which, it is said, will neutralise the geopathic stress in your home. There is also a small portable version of the RadiTech (TSP450), which is useful for travelling or for putting your feet on whilst working at an office desk. I realise that this takes a bit of believing, but it may not be as far-fetched as you might first think when you consider that radon gas, which occurs naturally in the ground, is thought to cause cancer and the incidence of leukaemia may be higher in children living close to electricity pylons. Certainly, since I took steps to rid myself of geopathic stress, I feel that I am responding to my therapies more effectively and I consider that it has played a crucial part in my recovery.

So do not dismiss this information – geopathic stress could be slowing your recovery. If you would like to know more about it, read *Are You Sleeping in a Safe Place?*, by Rolf Gordon (see page 177).

Electro-magnetic pollution may also have adverse effects on us. I couldn't even wear a battery-operated watch as it kept stopping!

Smoking

We are all aware how difficult it is for smokers to give up, even when they are full of good intentions and know the inherent dangers. But if you have M.E. and you do smoke, you should do your best to give up the habit.

Smoking interferes with your body's absorption of vital vitamins, like B and C; it is bad for the circulation; it may even aggravate irritable bowel problems. Recent research shows that smoking is particularly bad for the thyroid, which may already be functioning poorly.

Fortunately, help is at hand. Acupuncture has helped some people who really wanted to give up. There are brands of nicotine patches available from chemists, which, over a period of about three months, slowly reduce the craving for nicotine. They may cause side effects, like mouth ulcers or headaches, but some people find that they can give up smoking after only one month. The patches are expensive – but so are cigarettes. Herbal cigarettes are also available from health shops, which would keep idle hands safely occupied and away from other kinds.

If you do use patches, don't be tempted to sneak the odd fag too. There have been cases of fatalities, caused by the overload of nicotine.

Dental problems

Teeth are a bad enough problem when we are well, let alone when we have M.E.! When I have needed treatment and waited long enough for a spell of adequate energy to cope with it, I have found myself to be more than usually sensitive and have always needed an injection for a filling. Dental anaesthetic seems to have a very bad effect on me, however, and leads to a temporary setback. Different anaesthetics are available and it may be worth experimenting in case allergy causes an added problem. Adrenaline-free anaesthetic may also help; use Citanest. If at all possible, try to leave two or three months between appointments, so that your body can perk up again. It is a 'devil and the deep blue sea' situation and all I can do is to warn you about what might happen. Homoeopathic remedies such as arnica or hypericum may hasten your recovery.

I have just used hypericum 30 for the first time and got through the ordeal with no more than a headache. My energy level remained the same. I took one an hour before my treatment, one immediately afterwards and just one more a few hours on. Do consult your homoeopath. Through experience, I have discovered that longer visits and deeper drilling may require higher doses.

Mercury amalgam fillings

It has recently come to light from research that amalgam dental fillings may be adversely affecting many people.

I am not suggesting that removing amalgam fillings will be a miracle cure for M.E., but many sufferers become very sensitive and it could be another unwanted burden on their already weakened body. I personally know of someone who had migraines, together with food allergies, for over 20 years, and these disappeared as soon as four mercury amalgam fillings were removed.

When I first heard about these ideas some time ago, my first reaction was that it seemed a bit far-fetched that my fillings could be contributing to my bad health, but it seems possible that many people may be sensitive to mercury, which is twice as toxic as lead. After all, our teeth are part and parcel of our bodies. If they were not, they wouldn't hurt at the dentist. They are not just perched on top of our gums, they are connected to the bloodstream and nervous system. If I can be sensitive to wheat, I can surely be sensitive to mercury. Special homoeo-pathic drops are available which help to detoxify you of mercury. Some specialists in amalgam removal use Kelmer tablets or cysteine but you should only take these under specialist guidance. I have also tried D-Tox tablets, by Nutri Ltd, which seemed very effective, but are only available through a medical practitioner.

Germany has now banned amalgam fillings for pregnant women, children and people with kidney problems. Sweden has also started phasing them out altogether. Please note, however, that although it is possible to reduce mercury levels, they may rise again, so constant attention to your diet is necessary to keep them low. Some fish may be the culprit.

Removing amalgam fillings is difficult, due to the general state of the M.E. sufferer's health and the process will be very slow. All I can suggest is that every time you do manage to replace an old black filling, you have a white one. These are not suitable for all cavities, unfortunately. The other alternatives are crowns and porcelain inlays which are very expensive. I have avoided crowns as they involve gold and three other metals in the fixing procedure, and I would not recommend gold fillings as sensitivities could arise. Also, if you have a mixture of metals in your mouth, cross-currents of electrical activity can be set off, which is also bad for your health. My inlays are slowly falling to pieces but my fillings containing a strong glass component, which although were meant to be temporary, seem to be holding out quite well so far. There is now a new, cheaper and stronger form of inlay available – ask your dentist.

Now, only one more snag remains: when you have amalgam drilled out of your teeth, obviously some will finish up going down your throat, which we want to avoid. There is an answer to this: the dentist can fit a small rubber dam to your teeth, which acts as a shield and collects the fine powder. I couldn't see exactly how it was fitted as I was on the receiving end, but it wasn't a lot of bother. Talking is impossible, so arrange a bit of semaphore beforehand! A supplement of selenium could help counteract toxic effects and charcoal tablets will absorb any mercury which does find its way into your body.

Unfortunately, composite fillings do not last as well as amalgam, but I have heard of two which came highly recommended. One is called Nulite and the other Fuji 9, which is said to be self-curing (rather

61

like Araldite, I imagine) and sets almost as hard as amalgam.

Do beware however: amalgam removal can be difficult and dangerous to M.E. sufferers and should only be undertaken gradually over a long period of time with appropriate precautions.

Boosting the glandular system

When you have M.E., any part of your body can suffer, including your glandular system, which is vitally important to your health. The thyroid gland, which is situated in your neck, regulates your body's energy levels. The adrenal gland secretes a substance called hydrocortisone which has the effect of suppressing inflammatory reactions in the body and, to a lesser extent, the activities of the immune system. Malfunction of these glands can obviously cause symptoms very similar to M.E. Unfortunately, thyroid blood tests do not always give accurate results in M.E. sufferers.

If your temperature is consistently below 97.8°C first thing in the morning, this could indicate that you have a glandular problem. Take your temperature (three minutes under the tongue or ten minutes under your arm) before you get up. Incidentally, I have found that eating foods to which I am allergic also makes my temperature plummet.

Conventional treatment for malfunctioning thyroid and adrenals will include a course of thyroxine pills and hydrocortisone. These are both produced naturally by your body, but if you prefer, there are plenty of alternative remedies available to boost your glandular system. I avoid taking steroids at all costs as I believe that M.E. sufferers do not respond to them in the same way as 'normal' people. I have used Nature's Sunshine supplement Mastergland, which combines natural herbal products such as liquorice, alfalfa, kelp, ginseng and dong quai with essential minerals zinc, potassium and germanium. BioCare's TH207, for the thyroid, and AD206, for the adrenals, are also worth trying.

Please note, however, that anyone on hormone replacement therapy (HRT) should not take dong quai. Care should also be taken with kelp and iodine, which can be harmful in large quantities.

Travelling

At first, this will be out of the question if you are seriously ill. When you start to improve and feel like taking a little trip or holiday, let me give you a few words of warning: don't try to do too much; start with a short outing and see how you go and, as always with M.E., build up gradually.

Try going for short runs out in the car, being driven by a friend or family member. Make sure you can take frequent 'comfort' breaks and don't allow yourself to become hungry or thirsty. Just a few hours away from home will be quite enough to start with, so don't rush off for a long weekend when you haven't been out of the house for months. You'll end up exhausted and wishing you'd stayed at home in that prison you were so anxious to get out of!

63

Once you're on the road to recovery, flying abroad for a rest in the sun may sound marvellous but long-distance travel can exhaust M.E. sufferers. I could never understand why I slept for several days after my arrival abroad as all I had done was to sit in the car, sit in the plane and sit in the coach! However, my specialist explained that it is also the mental stress that wears us out. Just getting used to being in a strange environment can be wearing and in addition, subconsciously, we are wondering whether we will break down or miss the plane, whether the hotel will be all right, etc. It comes back to what I said earlier about mental stress being as tiring as physical stress.

There are physical problems too, of course. Carrying baggage and queuing are tiring and it is sometimes necessary to walk quite long distances. It may be sensible to arrange for a wheelchair for these emergencies. The worst problems are delays and night flights as there is nowhere to lie down.

I always enjoyed the rest in the sun once I got over the travelling, but needed another holiday when I got home again! However, if you feel you are in quite good nick, do give it a try. Remember to make your preparations gradually and early, check your medical insurance, make sure the local food is suitable and aim for somewhere healthy and safe so you don't need injections. Bear in mind that you will not have antibodies to foreign bugs. And, whatever you do, remember to rest and take things slowly.

Weather

Learning to adjust your lifestyle to the weather may help you deal with your illness. Many people find their problems improve in spring and summer, and deteriorate in autumn and winter. One reason may be the temperature, as M.E. sufferers always feel the cold and find warmth so relaxing. Also, more nasty viruses seem to abound in the winter, which pull us down badly and may aggravate any conditions we are already suffering from.

For M.E. sufferers with candida, it may be that the moulds associated with damp, wet or foggy days make them even worse. You should stay in a dry atmosphere if you can.

In the summer, there are longer hours of daylight, which when absorbed through our eyes (without glasses or contact lenses) will give us energy. We can get out to enjoy the fresh air more and oxygen is energising. Make the most of warm, sunny days.

However, do remember that we can also have humid days in the summer and there may be a lot of pollen and grass to contend with. Also, air conditioning may upset you with its icy blasts. Its humidity varies from 30 per cent to 70 per cent and M.E. sufferers are only really happy in the middle of that range.

You may even feel better in winter, in spite of the poor weather. I remember one summer when everything went completely wrong for me, followed by a good autumn and Christmas when I was free of viruses and using a new homoeopathy remedy.

Don't automatically expect to be worse for six months of the year and better for the next six. It won't necessarily happen like that!

Many people feel very disturbed when there are too few negative ions in the atmosphere, usually before a thunderstorm or at full moon. A shower of rain will create many negative ions, which is why you normally feel more refreshed after a shower than after a bath. Ionisers operate by creating thousands of negative ions. They vary in price and efficiency a great deal. The RadiTech (see page 57) improves air quality, and burning candles also increases the negative ions.

In winter when sunlight hours are short, you may find it helpful to use a lightbox (see page 183). These are designed for sufferers of the condition known as seasonal affective disorder (SAD), who become severely depressed by lack of natural sunlight. They should boost your energy levels as well as your flagging spirits. They are expensive, however, but you may find that a few daylight bulbs are a cheaper, helpful alternative.

CHAPTER 4

Allergies, Candida and Other Mouldy Conditions

If you are suffering from M.E., your immune system is out of balance. As a result, you are likely to suffer from exaggerated reactions by your immune system – allergies – to things which in most healthy people would cause no symptoms at all.

You will also be more prone to infection and, in particular, to a nasty fungal infection called candidiasis, or candida, for short.

M.E. is bad enough on its own but the additional misery of allergies and infections can make life really wretched at times. In this chapter, we shall look at these conditions and how you can control and reduce their effects.

Allergies

Allergies come in many forms: your skin, nose, lungs and digestive system can all become over-sensitive to substances around you. You may be allergic to things you touch, things you eat or things you breathe in the air. If you are suffering from geopathic stress, this will aggravate your allergic reactions and the outcome will be even more serious.

If you are allergic to something, the symptoms will arise very quickly: you may have itchy swellings or a rash; if your respiratory system is affected, you may suffer from sneezing, runny nose, sore itchy eyes and tight, difficult breathing; if your digestive system is sensitive to something you have eaten, you may suffer from diarrhoea or vomiting, tingling in the mouth or throat and lip swelling.

Allergic reactions come about for any number of reasons, such as candida, leaky gut, nutritional deficiency, unsuitable diet, antibiotics, infection, parasites, mercury overload, even eating too much of one thing. Avoiding the substances responsible, whether they be food, pollen, animal hair, chemicals, etc., will help your symptoms subside but first you will need to identify your problem areas. The most difficult may be food.

Cow's milk protein is a fairly common food allergy in young children but it also affects adults and other foods most commonly associated with allergies are wheat, fish (particularly shellfish) and eggs. In addition, many people are affected by yeast, corn, soya, nuts, citrus fruits, sugar and the potato family.

Other symptoms of intolerance may be headache, fatigue, joint pain, nausea, irritable bowel, even depression, anxiety and weight gain. If you decide to try elimination diets, it would be wise to have some good professional advice. When we eat a lot of a certain food, it can mask the fact that it is bad for us, but if we take it out of our diet for, say, two weeks and then eat it again, we will be in no doubt as to whether it upsets us or not. Never experiment with a food which you know you are sensitive to (for example, peanuts) or you may be made dangerously ill (e.g. with anaphylactic shock).

We have all used the expression 'a little of what you fancy does you good'. Where allergies are concerned forget it! People with allergies tend to crave the very things that most upset them. I can vouch for this. I would give my back teeth for a crusty roll, washed down with half a pint of sherry! However, from time to time, you should try a little nibble of your 'difficult', but healthy, foods just to see if they go down any better than they did a few weeks before.

Testing for allergies

Some people have used VEGA testing (see page 73), which has helped. This method, mostly available at private clinics, uses a machine which can test your sensitivity to many foods. Any sort of food testing will tell you if you are sensitive to a certain food *on that particular day*. The reliability of alternative methods of testing depends on the practitioner to a large extent. If you are sensitive to many foods, don't automatically drop them all in one go. Remember, some foods are likely to bother you much more than others, so try to work out a sensible compromise, perhaps rotating very mild problem foods every four to seven days. Trial and error will soon tell you what you can easily manage. Some people improve by eating just tiny amounts of the offending food, preferably with other foods rather than on their own.

Muscle testing (kinesiology)

I dare say some conventional doctors would gasp at this practice! However, it is used by many alternative practitioners and I have found it very accurate and generally used it to confirm my suspicions. It is done by holding the food in one hand, while the muscle power of the other arm is tested by your therapist. Offending foods instantly weaken the arm. On one occasion in London, I had just been tested for a food when a visiting doctor asked me if I would mind double-checking the result of the same food on his new machine that was being tried out. The result was absolutely identical. What was more surprising was that not only was an allergy detected in both cases, but the actual level of allergy to the same precise reading occurred in both cases.

Muscle testing can quite easily be learned if you have someone to show you, and practitioners of other therapies often learn it. Kinesiologists can do more for you than food allergy testing; see the address list at the back of the book for qualified practitioners.

Pulse testing

I have found this practice very useful too, but again many doctors would not give it credence.

Check your pulse rate before you start, then, about an hour after eating a suspect food, count your pulse rate over a minute and if it has gone up or down substantially (by about ten beats) this can indicate a problem. Before doing this, I made sure of what my normal pulse was by testing it several times a day for several days and discovered it was a constant 72. However, if your rate is very variable (even when you are not doing the hoovering!), then there is not much point in trying this exercise.

I never take one reading when food testing, but do it over and over again to make sure. I find that some foods regularly put it up a few beats (the ones that don't bother me too much) and others (the foods that give bad symptoms) will send it soaring or plummeting, with much higher or lower readings. Never test the same food more than once in a week.

Treatment for allergies

The simplest treatment for allergies of all kinds is avoiding the substance you are sensitive to – but first you have to know what it is! You can use one of the methods described above, or, if you prefer, your doctor can arrange for you to have patch tests for skin reactions, but food allergies are sometimes hard to establish. In fact, food intolerances often fail to register even in blood tests.

Conventional treatment consists of drugs, called anti-histamines, which relieve allergic symptoms, particularly the itching and sneezing. Many unfortunately have the effect of making you drowsy, but if you are very itchy this will help you to sleep. Many doctors also prescribe types of steroids which are normally very effective, but may cause very unpleasant side effects in M.E. sufferers. Make sure you discuss this very carefully with your doctor if he suggests either of these treatments. I cannot tolerate steroids at all but find that I can control my allergies successfully with natural alternative treatments and therapies.

Desensitising

It is possible to undergo desensitising treatments, which are particularly valuable for people who are allergic to insect bites, dust-mites or pollen. This is done by giving gradually increasing doses of the substance causing the allergic reaction, either by injection or by drops. Your body will then react by producing antibodies and these will then fight off future reactions.

Unfortunately, this treatment may produce mild side effects.

Knowing how sensitive I was, I was initially worried that this sort of treatment might make me worse as I had M.E. as well as allergies, so I put it off for three years. When I felt a bit stronger, I gave it a try for about seven weeks and I have to say that it made me decidedly worse, in spite of taking the drops at one-sixth of the normal dose (one every other day instead of three a day). The statistics at the clinic said that 90 per cent of their patients benefited from this treatment but my body was too ill and sensitive to withstand the cure! The unfortunate conclusion I drew was that the most ill and sensitive people may be the least likely to benefit.

I think that it is better to build up one's own health and immune system in a natural way, which in turn will make the body less sensitive eventually.

EPD is another form of desensitising, which involves injections of diluted food allergens mixed with an enzyme which are administered every few months. The therapy is expensive and usually available only through private clinics, the exception being the Royal Homoeopathic Hospital in London. It is said to have helped a number of people, but to date there are no proven results. I have not tried this treatment myself, but I understand that many people give up because of the unpleasant side effects they suffer.

However, the news on this front is not all gloomy. I was extremely fortunate to be treated by Mr Roger Rose who, in his retirement, specialised in the testing and treatment of all kinds using a VEGA machine. This mechanism can detect geopathic stress and the presence of viruses by measuring the way the body detects and reacts to stimuli from any given substance.

The method is quite simple and painless: the patient holds a simple electrode connected to the VEGA machine, while the operator places a measuring probe (not a needle), which is connected to the machine, on an acupuncture point on either a finger or a toe. Various substances, either animal, vegetable or mineral, depending on what is being investigated, are introduced into the machine and the results of the body's reaction to these substances are read on a meter. I found that it was very effective for testing for mercury toxicity, candida and geopathic stress.

Mr Rose was also an expert on the use of MORA therapy which helped with several of my problems.

MORA therapy was developed by a Dr Morelle and his son-in-law Erich Rasche, an electronic engineer (the machine gets its name from the first two letters of each of their names). Dr Morelle discovered that the oscillating electronic signals which are given off by all human tissue could be detected on the skin by using hand-held electrodes. Furthermore, he noticed that the signals from normal healthy tissue (which he referred to as 'harmonic') were different from those 'disharmonic' ones received from unhealthy tissue.

The MORA machine is able to identify these two different kinds of signal; it amplifies and reinforces the harmonic signals and reverses the disharmonic ones before returning them to the subject. The signals which have thus been reversed cancel out the original disharmonic signals and eventually eliminate the oscillations of the unhealthy tissue. This may all sound rather strange, but these principles are used in many other branches of physics!

MORA therapy is used to help to dislodge toxins and to balance the energies of the organs and bodily systems. Using these two methods, Mr Rose was able to discover the state of my immune system, whether I had any viral infection and what parasites I was harbouring; he treated me most successfully with his homoeopathic remedies which worked wonders for me. Best of all, it meant I did not have to take antibiotics, which make me ill. His remedies have not given me any problems and my troubles are fading. Mr. Rose also uses electro-acupuncture (which does not involve the use of needles).

Unfortunately, my allergies have proved to be very stubborn although a few improvements have occurred of their own accord. It would seem that some people, who have been very ill with multiple problems, are difficult to treat.

Candida

As well as allergies, M.E. sufferers seem very prone to candida, or candidiasis, to give it its full name.

Candida is caused by *candida albicans*, a very small yeasty organism, which lives in everyone's bowel and intestines along with many other organisms. It belongs to the same family as mushrooms and moulds, and normally it is kept under control by bacteria present in our body. However, if these bacteria are destroyed, it gets out of control and invades parts of the body where it isn't welcome. After a while, it can reach a level where it changes its form and literally grows little legs, which burrow into our gut. It is now literally a deep-rooted problem and a difficult parasite to get rid of.

The two commonest causes of candida are: firstly, the weakening of your immune system by illness (so it is common amongst sufferers of AIDS as well as M.E.); and secondly, overuse of antibiotics which unbalance your body's natural defence system. Antibiotics can be a boon for serious illnesses, but if they are taken too often, they will destroy the 'good' bacteria inside us as well as the 'baddies'. For this reason, they are seldom suitable for M.E. sufferers who have so many recurrent problems.

Oral contraceptives, which may upset the bacterial balance of the vagina and interfere with our hormones, may also aggravate candida, so women who suffer may be advised to change to a non-hormonal method of contraception.

Stress, poor diet, pollution and diabetes may also be involved in encouraging candida.

Candida may spread to other moist areas of the body including the mouth, bowel, digestive tract, vagina and even the skin.

It is easy to see candida (or thrush as it is sometimes called) on the tongue or in the form of a creamy vaginal discharge. The discharge is white or yellow and may lead to itchiness and soreness. Olive oil on cotton wool can be used to clean any sensitive areas, and tea tree oil may be put in the bath. Never try to scrub the nasty stuff away. Although a vaginal discharge in M.E. sufferers is very likely to be candida, it could be something else. If in doubt, check with your doctor.

Candida and your diet

Most candida sufferers are intolerant of yeast, and diets high in sugar and refined starchy food will also worsen the condition. Fermented substances like alcohol and vinegar should be avoided too. Plenty of fibre will help to blot up the toxins and lots of fresh water will swill them through. Try to eat only fresh food and avoid all artificial additives, including sweeteners. For further information, see the chapter on food and diet.

Helping your body to get rid of candida

Getting rid of candida if you are a normal, healthy person can be difficult and take time, so in M.E. sufferers, who have an abnormal immune system, it can take absolutely ages. However, do not despair. I did start to feel some benefits quite early on, although I have still not finished the job some years later! My main improvement at first was relief from constant indigestion, but it took longer to get to the real roots of the problem. Eventually, homoeopathic drops speeded things up.

Magazines and advertisements will inform you that in order to rid yourself of thrush, all you have to do is wear loose clothing, avoid bubble bath and use a particular product! Unfortunately, it is not usually that simple. The visible symptoms of thrush can be just a sign that there are worse things going on inside. It is only by treating your digestive system and health as a whole that you will be able to get control over this nuisance. If you don't, you are likely to feel more and more ill. Many people have noticed that their health improves overall when they pay more particular attention to their insides. Just think how dismal you feel all over when your tummy is upset.

There are lots of things we can do to help get rid of candida. Diet is very important but not usually enough just by itself.

Antifungal drugs

The most commonly used are Nystatin, Fungalin and Amphotericin B. There is no doubt that some people have benefited from them, but they are most effective when used to treat the *early* stages of candida before it 'digs in'.

The first time I took Nystatin, it made such a big difference that I thought I was starting to recover from M.E. The lethargy started disappearing for the first time in nearly 18 months. Unfortunately, this didn't last for long and when I had some more a bit later on, the effect was somewhat less strong. The third lot seemed finally to help me only when I was on holiday and resting literally every day on a sunbed. On reflection, I think it was probably the rest that did me good.

Some doctors do not agree with antifungal drugs for a number of reasons: once the candida has taken a firm grip and become systemic, taking drugs just wipes away the top layer of the candida and leaves the roots to thrive, just like a lawn mower taking off the top of the grass and leaving the grass to grow back even more strongly. Also, there is more than one strain of candida, so one drug cannot properly get rid of the whole problem.

Some doctors regard these drugs as unsafe when they have the chance to seep through the leaky gut into the bloodstream and possibly damage the liver. Others think they cannot work properly unless they actually do get into the bloodstream!

It is now suspected that Nystatin may also kill off good bacteria and possibly vitamin B_2 and B_6, which are very important.

Natural supplements

If you are unhappy about taking antifungal drugs, there are some natural supplements which may be of benefit to you.

Garlic is one of nature's best antibiotics. It is best eaten fresh and in cooking, but can be supplemented with capsules as well. These are best taken at night or on their own, but to minimise digestive problems, take them after food. Over-consumption of garlic will wipe out the goodies as well as the baddies.

Biocidin Forte (grapefruit seed concentrate) is a naturally based supplement which may help you fight your candida as well as parasite invaders.

Caprylic acid is a natural product made from coconuts, which is effective in destroying yeasts. Capricin is a good make as it releases slowly and has a chance to reach as far as the bowel. I have had the best results with Micopryl 680 from BioCare, which disperses well into all the parts the other pills don't reach!

Lactobacillus acidophilus and **bifidus** are two good bacteria which live in our gut and bowel. Bifidus can be found in brands of live yoghurt such as Loseley BA. Taking caprylic acid and acidophilus together on a regular basis can make quite a difference. Never use tap water to take acidophilus as the chlorine kills all bugs, good and bad alike. Replete, by BioCare, is expensive (about £30 for a week's supply) but contains generous amounts of acidophilus, bulgaricus and bifidus. It provides a good boost for anyone with a candida problem.

Pau D'Arco / Taheebo tea is a natural product made from a tree bark and has good antifungal properties. It is expensive and may not be easily tolerated by those M.E. sufferers having trouble with tea and herbal tea already, but worth a try. It can also be purchased in tablet form.

Aloe vera comes in the form of cream, ointment or drink. The drink is good for helping to heal a 'leaky gut' caused by candida. Brands vary enormously in quality.

Cold-pressed olive oil contains **oleic acid**, which is effective against candida. It is a good idea to drizzle it over your salads. Olive oil also contains **butyric acid**, which is good for the bowel.

Vitamins and minerals will help boost the immune system in general, along with a healthy and nutritious diet. By and large, the supplements will be the same as those required to help your M.E. Evening primrose oil, zinc and selenium are all said to be particularly helpful.

Avoiding mould

Moulds are in the same family as yeasts and it helps to avoid these. They lurk in the most unexpected places. Moulds thrive in dark, damp areas and hate light and dry air. Watch out for trouble spots such as the bathroom, in the corners low down, or on grouting between tiles; kitchens, on tile grouting, around the sink, behind taps, etc.; damp cupboards (especially overloaded ones which do not leave room for air to circulate); old newspapers, books or leather; decaying vegetation, such as old vegetables or house plants, whose earth can get mouldy too; compost heaps, grass cuttings; even cold, damp buildings, like churches in winter, play havoc with my nose! Keep all bedding, upholstery and carpets as clean as possible.

Chemical and perfume allergies

Chemical and perfume allergies often become much stronger with M.E. and avoidance of these, as far as possible, will take a weight off your immune system. Below is a list of the more common problem products: many of them contain petroleum.

Gas fumes	Petrol fumes
Cleaning fluids	Bleach
Ammonia	Turpentine
Shoe polish	Marker pens
Cleaning sprays	Air fresheners
Paint	Rubber
Plastic	Man-made textiles
Nail varnish	Cosmetics
Soap	Hairspray
Perfume, after-shave	Tobacco smoke

Any house needs to be ventilated from time to time to get rid of the build-up of toxic air. The kitchen probably collects more, because of the number of cleaning materials and gas cooking, and needs the window open as much as possible. You can improve on your cleaning materials – soap, hand cream, etc. – by buying unperfumed varieties. Also, Ecover make good washing-up liquid, bleach, etc., which are safer alternatives for you and the environment. I also prefer to use non-scented/non-biological detergents, from Marks & Spencer, which have the added advantage of not clogging up my washing machine.

It is worth noting that people with multiple chemical sensitivities and organo-phosphate poisoning show strong M.E.-type symptoms.

CHAPTER 5

Treatment

Many doctors will admit that they are baffled by M.E: the sheer number of symptoms presented by sufferers seems to be outnumbered only by the combinations in which they present themselves!

It is generally accepted, however, that M.E. is an abnormal reaction by the body to some kind of stress, very often accompanied by a viral 'trigger'. Identifying the source of the stress is helpful as a starting point for treatment, but finding effective, all-round treatment for all those symptoms can be a nightmare, and curing the patient altogether may prove impossible.

There are two kinds of treatment available for any illness: conventional treatment, which is what you get from your family doctor; and alternative therapies, which include any medical system based on a theory of disease or method of treatment other than the orthodox science of medicine as it is taught in our medical schools. These therapies include, amongst others, homoeopathy, reflexology, aroma-therapy and chiropractic.

Not surprisingly, because M.E. has such a large number of different aspects to it, many sufferers try a combination of both conventional and alternative treatments. What may surprise you more is the number of doctors who actually encourage the use of alternative therapies. Some, such as acupuncture and homoeopathy, are actually available, to a limited degree, on the NHS.

In this chapter, we shall look at both kinds of treatment and the most effective therapies they offer for the M.E. sufferer.

The process of diagnosis

Let's start with your doctor – as you probably will. When you first go to your doctor with your (long) list of symptoms, it is highly unlikely that she will say 'Yes, of course, you have got M.E.'. It is not just that simple and, as we have already seen, the symptoms of M.E. overlap with those of many other conditions. So it is important that you do not jump to any conclusions until she has been through the full diagnostic process.

In order to assess your particular condition, the first thing your doctor will probably do is give you a full physical examination. She may take a sample of blood; this is a bit like an initial full body screening. Tests on this can reveal many things, for example, evidence of bowel disorders, kidney disease, liver malfunction and even any past or current infection you may have suffered.

If you are presenting obvious symptoms, such as a urinary infection or a severe cough, she may arrange for further investigations, including X-rays, if she feels this is necessary.

She may ask you questions about your lifestyle, any recent changes in your career or home situation, any illnesses you may have suffered recently, even about your relationships. Some of these questions may seem rather strange, but if she suspects you have M.E., she will be looking for the stress factor, or factors, that triggered it.

Symptomatic treatment

If you have a sore throat, a terrible hacking cough, constipation, or indeed any obvious physical complaint, she will certainly try to treat these first. Do not think she is trying to fob you off: she may or may not think you have M.E., but she is trying to build up a full picture of your illness in order to make an accurate diagnosis and it is important to treat all the possible minor ailments first. After all, not everyone with a persistent sore throat has M.E. So you may come away from your visit with a prescription for antibiotics.

If they clear up your symptoms and you feel better, then you obviously do not have M.E. and that will be the end of it. If, however, those symptoms clear up but you still feel ill, or experience other symptoms, then the investigation and elimination process must go on.

The doctor may refer you for other treatment, such as physiotherapy, or, if she thinks the cause of your illness may be stress-related, then she may refer you for counselling.

Counselling

At this point, many of you think you are being labelled as a mentally unstable malingerer. This is NOT the case.

As I have already said, it is well established that most doctors believe that M.E. is caused or preceded by stress, which may be physical (for example, injury or illness) or emotional (overwork, change of school or bereavement). If you are to overcome M.E., you will first have to identify the source of your stress and then perhaps change your lifestyle to accommodate it. Both of these take a great deal of time.

Counsellors have both the time to talk to sufferers and the skills to understand their problems. Their expertise may be invaluable in getting you back on your feet and able to live life normally again. So, once again, please don't be put off, don't be offended. Your counsellor may help you change your life, for the better.

One method commonly used is called cognitive behavioural therapy. This is a specialised form of counselling based on the idea that the way we perceive the world and ourselves (our cognition) influences our emotions and behaviour. The therapy focuses on the here and now, rather than the past; it aims to help clients find new positive ways of thinking and encourages them to try out new ideas in their everyday activities. It is direct, individual, structured and active. Ideas and suggestions are thrown about and those which seem relevant are put into practice. In due course, as the mental attitude

86

changes, the body follows suit and physical improvements will be made.

No pressure is put on the client to do more than is possible, but improvement can be the natural outcome. I myself know of someone who was so ill, she could only lie in bed; within a few weeks of receiving two weeks' cognitive behavioural therapy in hospital, she was able to go for a walk.

Once again, I will stress, however, that I do not think that M.E. is a mental illness, but simply that the mind is involved in any illness. For some people, perhaps, this mental therapy gives the lift-off required to start the journey towards recovery.

Looking for the cure

I have spoken about symptomatic treatment already – that is, the treatment the doctor gives you to relieve the misery of all those sore throats, aching limbs, headaches, constipation, sleeplessness and so on. If you have M.E., however, this relief does not constitute a cure. Unfortunately, much of the treatment for M.E., whether it is conventional or alternative, is purely symptomatic. The cure is more likely to lie in the process of removing the stresses that caused it in the first place.

All sorts of treatment

Let's look now at the treatments which are available to M.E. sufferers. There are literally dozens and there is no way of telling which may be best for you.

It really is a matter of trial and error, horses for courses, whatever you like to call it. I can only say that I wish I had discovered homoeopathy sooner – it has worked wonders for me. Remember, any symptomatic treatment, conventional or alternative, which gives you relief is a good thing. Relief brings freedom from stress and with it, the road to recovery.

Prescribed drugs

There is a long list of drugs commonly prescribed for the symptoms presented by sufferers of M.E. It includes antibiotics; anti-inflammatories; steroids; betablockers (for excessive sweating, palpitations and trembling muscles); sleeping tablets; painkillers; tricyclic antidepressants; tranquillisers and SSRIs (for example, Prozac).

These are all effective treatments in the appropriate circumstances but I have to say that I did not benefit from any conventional medication and I do not believe that these drugs are suitable for M.E. sufferers. In my opinion, they worsen your condition – even over-the-counter medicines upset some of us. I would particularly avoid taking Prozac or steroids, so if your doctor offers you these, do ask about their side effects.

For me, real relief and improvement were found through alternative natural remedies and complementary therapies.

I found excellent alternatives in natural remedies and homoeopathy: for example, Efamol Marine, which contains primrose oil and fish oil, is a safe alternative to conventional anti-inflammatories; KIRA tablets, which contain the herb hypericum, are effective antidepressants; Bach Flower Rescue Remedy is an excellent calming alternative to tranquillisers; health shops sell good cough mixtures made from natural ingredients; and vitamin C, echinacea, garlic and propolis can all be used to ward off infections.

Gammaglobulin injections

These may be offered to help boost the immune system. These are given in the muscle, and may cause unpleasant side effects. I was offered these, but changed my mind as I considered them to be foreign bodies that would make me ill.

Magnesium injections

In the early 1990s, Southampton University claimed that magnesium could make a big difference to M.E. sufferers if administered by injection. Immediately, sufferers everywhere were demanding injections from their doctors, thinking there might be a magic cure at last. Unfortunately not. Not all sufferers are low in magnesium and too much magnesium in itself can be dangerous.

Injections should not be given if there are indications of any heart or kidney troubles. It is essential to make sure you are definitely deficient in magnesium before considering them and this is not as easy as it sounds. Some doctors and hospitals are unwilling to administer the blood tests and some doctors will not give the injections, although they are available on the NHS.

It is now accepted that only red blood cell magnesium gives an accurate picture but you may need to go to BioLab in London for an accurate red blood cell magnesium test. In carefully conducted study trials, 80 per cent of participants, who were deemed to be low in magnesium improved. Blood testing for magnesium deficiency is carried out at various hospital pathology labs.

Possible signs of lack of magnesium are muscle weakness, pain, cold hands and feet, twitching, constipation, palpitations, loss of appetite, general fatigue, dizziness, insomnia and numbness and tingling: all, in fact, common M.E. symptoms.

If you do embark on this course of action, make absolutely sure that you are under the care of a medically qualified practitioner. Please note that these injections of magnesium sulphate must be administered into a muscle (bumjabs!), and not intravenously (in the vein), which could be dangerous for the heart and kidneys.

Magnesium can be taken by mouth as a supplement and is available from BioCare in a more absorbable form, called Bio-magnesium or magnesium EAP. It is also available from Solgar combined with calcium and boron (good for the bones). Most people try taking it orally first, but there are some seriously ill people who may well be 'sieving' out all their magnesium which is a very serious condition indeed. It is probably these people who have responded well to tiny amounts of magnesium being administered by injection.

Opinions on the effectiveness of this treatment are divided and they certainly do not suit everyone, but I think if I were in a wheelchair with the classic symptoms of deficiency and a blood test to confirm this, I would be tempted to risk one or two of these injections and see what happened.

Foods which contain magnesium are green salads, green vegetables, nuts, beans, soya beans, lentils, wholegrains, fish, prawns, meat and milk.

Action for M.E. have a 'Magnesium Pack', which gives full information on testing for deficiency and administering the treatment (not for you to use!), price £1.50 to practitioners and members. There is also a general fact sheet on magnesium, which you may find useful.

Complementary Therapy

Complementary therapy is particularly suitable for M.E. sufferers as the therapists treat patients in an holistic way, i.e. trying to help the whole person to regain a balance within their body by seeking out the root cause of the problem rather than simply relying on symptomatic treatment. When considering alternative therapies, however, it is a good idea not to mix too many at the same time as I think that your body could become over-stimulated and the immune system confused.

Always choose a qualified, registered practitioner (see list on pages 180–1).

Drawing from my own experience only, I would

suggest the following guidelines:

Homoeopathy (see pages 99–101) stands well alone but mixes well with herbal medicine.

Acupuncture (see pages 93–5) and herbal medicine mix well (as any Chinese will tell you).

The Bowen Technique (see pages 96–8) has to be taken alone, away from other hands-on therapies, although I safely continued with homoeopathy.

Reflexology (see pages 110–111) causes no problems when combined with homoeopathic remedies.

Massage (see pages 104–7) is often too strong for M.E. sufferers, but if it can be tolerated, it is wonderful.

Aromatherapy (see page 96) may upset sufferers who cannot bear the effect of the essential oils.

Lymphatic drainage massage (see pages 102–4) requires about ten initial sessions, so I took no other therapies except my homoeopathy at that time.

Magnetic therapy (see pages 101–3), I have found, can be used continuously and I have undergone Christian healing or Reiki daily.

Physiotherapy, Alexander technique, osteopathy and cranio-sacral therapy I feel would mix with anything except Bowen Technique.

Acupuncture

We have all heard of acupuncture, but how many of us know what it is used for or roughly how it works? In fact, it can be used on almost everybody for very many conditions and produces good results, though these will obviously vary from person to person. Even conventional doctors are tending to accept and recommend it more now.

There is some mystery as to exactly how it works but the basic principles are as follows: the body has 14 meridians (channels) through which our energy flows. The Chinese call this current of energy 'Chi' and consider it to be our vital force. Think of it as your 'get-up-and-go'. When you have plenty of it, you feel pretty well, don't you? By stimulating these channels at specific points (acupoints), blocked energy can be released and health restored. Acupuncture puts the body back in balance. These meridians carry energy to all your important organs, so it is thought that acupuncture treats the whole body and helps to build up your immune system. Insertion of needles also helps the brain to release endorphins (the body's natural painkillers).

Acupuncture needles are very fine and cause little discomfort – a quick pin-prick, but nothing like an injection. You are unlikely to have more than eight or ten needles, which are in before you know it, and then you can relax.

Acupuncture uses needles, but other methods of application are available, which include acupressure (massage on the acupoints), electrical stimulation, heat and lasers. These methods are preferable for people who do not like needles.

There are few side effects of acupuncture, the main one being that you may feel worse for a few days before you feel better. This is quite normal with alternative medicine and is considered to be a good sign. This 'healing crisis', as it is called, means that you are benefiting from the treatment. Possible side effects after early treatments are tiredness, sweating, loose bowels, skin irritation or an apparent cold. These do not last long. I felt as if I had a cold and was rather tired, but that was all.

It is a good idea to have a rest when you get home for maximum benefit. This is not usually difficult as acupuncture tends to have a relaxing effect on most people.

The method of diagnosis used by acupuncturists is very interesting. Your therapist will tell a lot from your tongue and your pulses. I always thought we had only one pulse, but apparently we have twelve, six on each wrist. Each one can be felt separately and according to the strength of the beat, your therapist can tell which organs need a bit of a boost.

If you decide to try acupuncture, make sure you find a well qualified therapist (see the address list at the back of the book). Most professional treatments cost around £20–£30 per session.

Some experienced Chinese therapists combine acupuncture with herbal medicine and sometimes other alternative medicine; I have heard good reports of their results with M.E. sufferers.

Some chartered physiotherapists have also trained in acupuncture. All chartered physiotherapists using acupuncture are trained to give pain relief, but extra training is required to treat complex problems like M.E. As you can imagine, this treatment is not widely available on the NHS but it is worth enquiring at your local hospital if private treatment is too expensive.

If you attend a physiotherapist/acupuncturist, you should be offered the added benefits of relaxation techniques, help with hyperventilation, breathing exercises, pain relief of the neck, etc. and perhaps later on, some very gentle exercises to do at home, when you are a lot better.

Acupuncture is not a magic wand for curing M.E. but, combined with other sensible management, it can help build up your immune system. I personally know of two people who responded to it so well that they had virtually recovered in a year, but one was combined with herbal treatment and the other homoeopathic remedies. The effects have not been quite so dramatic for me, but it has generally and slowly improved my level of health; it has pulled me out of the black hole when I have been very ill with viruses; it has probably helped to keep me from being permanently confined to a wheelchair.

Acupuncture is a good but slow therapy; the effects accumulate over time. It can take several months for a seriously ill person to feel any benefit but if you are prepared to be patient, I would still recommend it.

Aromatherapy

This form of massage has become very popular recently, but M.E. sufferers should be wary: it should not be considered until you are virtually well. Do bear in mind that it is not just massage, but a strong form of medicine that uses the beneficial properties of plant essences, and care needs to be taken with sensitive people. Personally, I cannot tolerate the oils, which give me a thumping headache and upset my nose. However, many people enjoy the positive benefits of aromatherapy, and a qualified therapist should be able to advise you on the choice of oils.

Body brushing

Like massage, body brushing eliminates toxins and aids circulation but, unlike massage, you can do it yourself. Don't attempt it if you have sore, tender muscles. The bristle brushes, available at places like The Body Shop, are not as hard as you might imagine, but, alternatively, you could use a rough flannel or massage sponge, which would be more gentle. Start at the feet and always work up the limbs towards the heart, using short, overlapping strokes of the brush. Make the session short and light: don't turn it into a long massage.

The Bowen Technique

This technique only arrived in Britain in 1993, so you may not have heard of it. Tom Bowen took many years to develop this therapy, which helped thousands of people in Australia and is now showing favourable results with M.E. here.

It is quite different from anything else I have ever tried and involves the precise manipulation of muscle and connective tissue, which stimulates your energy to flow. It helps circulation, lymphatic drainage, assimilation of nutrients, elimination of toxins and joint mobility. It has been used a great deal for sporting injuries but it is equally effective for migraine, asthma, hay fever, organic diseases, bronchial conditions, stress and tension. Because it taps into the body's natural healing response, it doesn't matter what is wrong, it could help *you*.

I recently had a series of treatments using this technique; a month was enough before a break was required. I actually felt heat being released through my back as the energy started to flow.

During the second two weeks of treatment, I also had a RadiTech installed (see page 57), which I feel made a lot of difference to the way in which I responded to my therapies, especially homoeopathy. During this time, my energy levels improved significantly, whilst my lower back pain was reduced.

There are currently only around 300 Bowen Technique therapists in the country, but I feel this will grow in popularity and be more readily available in the future.

I have just had a second session of four treatments and have to say that my last two weeks have been my best ever. Although I know that homoeopathy is still my main support, I do feel that the Bowen

Technique has been a real bonus. From what I hear, many patients respond even more quickly than I have. This is not a therapy that goes on indefinitely: it either helps or it doesn't – and mostly it does. At about £15 a session, it is reasonably priced compared with other therapies.

Colonic irrigation

Colonic irrigation is the official term for a whopping enema! The idea behind washing out the colon is to get rid of the conglomeration of rubbish that accumulates there, like dead yeast cells, viruses and old muck that has hardened and glued itself to the wall. This sounds all right in theory but many doctors think it is rather violent and even positively dangerous, as there is a danger of perforation under the water pressure. If it is ever undertaken, it must be done by an expert.

This treatment is unsuitable for sufferers of some conditions, including high blood pressure. Some critics also say that after all the debris is washed away, the good bacteria are washed away too, and must be replaced artificially. Others claim that until the colon is cleaned up, it won't function properly anyway and there won't be anything to waste!

However, there are alternative and gentler ways of spring-cleaning our interiors and ensuring regular bowel movements. Health shops and mail order companies sell products such as psyllium husks, herbal tablets and olive oil cream. Even body brushing may help through its stimulating effect on the circulation. A healthy, balanced diet with plenty of fibre is essential for everyone, but especially for M.E. sufferers.

Foods high in fibre such as fruit and vegetables have excellent cleansing properties. Alfalfa and chlorophyll supplements could be useful too.

Homoeopathy

This is currently proving to be the therapy most helpful to me and I wish I had understood more about it earlier. I used to think it meant mixing up herbal cough mixture instead of buying it from the chemist! It is, in fact, a simple form of medicine, which requires long study just like conventional medicine. The difference is that homoeopathy treats the whole of the body and mind and uses 'safe', natural remedies instead of artificial drugs. It has been proved that adults, children and even animals can all benefit from homoeopathic treatment.

Benefit can only be derived if accurate diagnosis is made and this is quite a lengthy affair, requiring long appointments during which the patient's medical history, present state of health and much more will be assessed and recorded. It is up to the patient to answer questions as fully as possible in order to help the homoeopath come to the correct conclusions. All the questions have a purpose.

This holistic therapy (treating the whole body and mind) has been around for 200 years and really gets to the roots of the illness, enabling the sick to regain good health slowly and completely. Your physical, mental, emotional and even spiritual problems are all closely connected and all affect the progress of your illness. In order to heal, all these must be taken into account when prescribing remedies. M.E. is quite a challenge for a homoeopath!

Your first consultation could take up to two hours and will be the most expensive (about £40–£45). After that, further consultations to discuss progress and possibly modify remedies as time goes by will be at roughly two-monthly intervals and less costly (around £25–£30 a time). Homoeopathic treatment can be slow to get going and there are over 2,000 remedies to choose from! However, it is worth being patient as even very slow progress is better than none at all and M.E. sufferers' health can remain unimproved for months on end.

There is very little homoeopathy available under the NHS. If you don't know of a suitable practitioner or the cost is prohibitive, your doctor may be able to refer you on the NHS to the Royal Homoeopathic Hospital at Great Ormond Street in London. They are very good with M.E. and provide you with transport. If your doctor is uncooperative, get in touch with the Society of Homoeopaths (see page 180) for advice.

Remedies are made from plants, minerals, metals and even poisons, but all are perfectly safe to take as long as you are under expert supervision. This means you must find a registered and qualified homoeopath (see address list at back of book). The base material used to make these little pills has been diluted hundreds of times and shaken between each dilution. In fact, in the end, there is no measurable trace of the original material left: I was certainly glad of this when taking arsenic!

However, the healing energy is still there and still works. Their strength lies in their weakness. No one quite fully understands *exactly* how they nudge your immune system into action, but they do. The natural medicine works with your body and stimulates your immune system to get on with the job of healing itself.

Homoeopathic remedies work on a 'like-for-like' principle. The remedy matches the symptoms. That is the meaning of the word homoeopathy (it is based on the Greek for 'similar suffering'). To take an easy example – if you were feverishly hot, you would not be given something cold to cool you down, but rather something hot. This seems to neutralise the problem.

There are no nasty side effects, but you may feel worse just for a day or so after taking a new pill. This is a actually a good sign and means the remedy should help, so do not be put off.

You may also be interested to know that all the remedies have been tested on human volunteers over the years and not on animals.

Magnetic therapy

The beneficial effects of magnetism on the body have been known for over 400 years.

One of the problems of the twentieth century is that

we are not getting enough magnetic radiation. This is compounded by too many electro-magnetic fields from electrical equipment and domestic appliances. We spend too much time in concrete buildings, planes and cars, and not enough time outside in the fresh air.

Nikken produce many magnetic products which may redress this imbalance. Magnetic therapy works by homing in on the iron in the blood, setting up a whirlpool effect and sending the blood coursing more efficiently round the body with all its attendant benefits. Blood is not called life blood for nothing.

Two of their popular products are inner soles for your shoes and a seat cover, which can double as a mattress. I certainly had a strange night the first time I slept on the cover. I woke up several times feeling hot and restless and my body felt very busy. The next day I felt very tired, but after that I think I slept even better. It is hard to assess the short-term benefits for something new like this, but I certainly got over my second dose of flu very well. I also find it very warming to lie on after about 40 minutes.

The MagneTech, produced by Dulwich Health, is a machine first invented to eliminate mercury from the body (denture amalgam). The following are some of the aspects which may be helped in M.E. sufferers: back injury, tinnitus (if combined with osteopathy and a careful diet), joint pain, toxins, sore muscles, food allergy, poor circulation, disorders of the colon, hiatus hernia, irritable bowel, low energy, weakened immune system and hypoglycaemia.

Very full details of this therapy are available from Rolf Gordon at Dulwich Health.

I recently purchased a MagneTech and am delighted at how much it has helped my really bad shoulder, which did not respond to physiotherapy or acupuncture. I can now write and peel vegetables again. I also think that, along with homoeopathic drops, it has helped reduce my mercury levels.

Manual lymphatic drainage

The lymphatic system works in close conjunction with the immune system, so if either of these is low, it is likely to pull the other one down below par. Anything which improves the efficiency of your lymphatic system may boost your immune system.

A series of ten manual lymphatic drainage treatments would be ideal, the earlier ones being close together and the later ones more spread out. The movements are soft and rhythmic and counted in multiples of five. The areas worked on can include the head and face, and always the neck; chest, stomach, legs, feet, buttocks, lower, middle and upper back, shoulders, arms and hands. If all these were done in one session, it would take all of two hours and probably be too much, too soon for the client. Usually an hour is enough and different areas can be selected according to individual needs at different sessions.

I certainly felt these were doing me good and made some improvement. There were small signs of a healing crisis (a good sign that it is working), such as sudden severe headaches, eruption of a few spots and pain under the armpits.

It is essential to drink plenty of water after these sessions to help eliminate toxins – about two litres a day, or possibly more.

Massage

Massage is a controversial topic: one book will tell you it is good for M.E. and another will tell you it is bad. After a lot of recent investigation, I have come to the conclusion that, like so many treatments, it is a matter of horses for courses!

In healthy people, it can have enormous benefits in relieving tension and thereby inducing relaxation and pain relief. However, M.E. is a large umbrella covering many types of people with many types of problems, and among these there will be some who will be made ill by massage and others who will need it as part of their treatment for back problems.

If you decide to try it, be sure that you go to an experienced and qualified physiotherapist who has knowledge of the needs of M.E. sufferers. Your doctor or local health shop may help you find one, or someone you know may be able to recommend a good one they have tried. Whatever you do, don't go for a full body massage at your local beauty salon!

Massage is best left to the experts at first but when you are virtually better, it could be a good way of keeping relaxed, enjoying yourself and maintaining good health.

However, you will have to be well on the way to recovery before you can even consider it, as massaging a sore, tender or painful body could make it even worse and you would not even enjoy it if you felt really poorly. However, when you start to make good progress, and provided your body is comfortable to touch, a *gentle* massage will feel lovely and do you good. M.E. sufferers may especially feel the benefit of massage around the neck and shoulders, which become so tight and stiff.

You should have a relaxing massage, certainly not an invigorating one. Do not even consider very firm pressure at first, or those chopping movements you always see on the telly! When this once accidentally happened to me, I felt ill for days and it really hurt my calves, which hadn't bothered me much until they were walloped!

Your therapist will be trained to recognise certain conditions that are not suitable for massage, but may not know a lot about M.E. It will be helpful if you explain your problems and thereby get the best possible treatment.

Do not have a massage if you suffer from any of the following:

Sore, tender muscles	Rashes
Inflammation	Bruising
Eczema	Broken bones
Varicose veins	Fever
Swellings or tumours	Thrombosis problems
Kidney disease	Cancer
Pregnancy	Back injury with oedema

M.E. sufferers with back problems should be particularly wary of massage. There is a school of thought that suggests that the depleted state we call M.E. may be the result of an old back injury, not necessarily a severe one.

In his book *The Back and Beyond*, Dr Paul Sherwood explains that a back injury may damage the ability of surrounding muscles to pump blood efficiently. As a result, oedema (waterlogging) builds up in the tissues, preventing the parasympathetic nervous system from working properly. This gives rise to symptoms typical of M.E.

Along similar lines, Raymond Perrin, a Manchester osteopath, first became aware of the link between M.E. and back problems in 1989. He spent many years investigating the potential link before beginning a research programme, with clinical trials, at the Department of Orthopaedic Mechanics at the University of Salford.

He recognises that many M.E. sufferers have mechanical and postural defects, even though they may be totally unaware of it and suffering no back pain. Their problems can affect the sympathetic nervous system, which in turn is linked to the lymphatic system; if these are not functioning correctly, a vicious circle of events ensues, which we recognise as M.E. A charity called FORME has been set up to fund the research (see page 180). Osteopaths can obtain step-by-step technique information free of charge; others will have to pay a small administration charge.

Sufferers with a suspected back injury should therefore avoid massage, as, although it may give initial relief, it may aggravate the waterlogging.

If you think you have a back injury associated with M.E., you should go to a qualified physiotherapist or osteopath who will be able to feel if you have a muscle spasm over your back and may use treatments such as manipulation, surged faradism (a sort of electrical massage) or ultrasound.

If you have a broken bone or patches of eczema, limited massage may still be given. If you are in any doubt, consult your doctor first.

Massage is beneficial in two ways: firstly, it helps the elimination and drainage of toxins (poisons). (I am sure we have plenty of those to get rid of!) Secondly, it is also good for circulation, tension, stress and even pain. By taking the tension out of muscles, massage eases pain and fatigue and induces rest and relaxation.

Some practitioners use a gently vibrating bed. It relaxes the patient and helps joint pain and circulation problems.

Oxygen therapy

Oxygen is vital to our very existence. It cleanses and detoxifies our bodies and keeps us healthy. Unfortunately, we are not getting as much as we used to, due to polluted air. Shallow breathing, stress and lack of exercise make the problem worse. Therefore, we accumulate in our systems waste products, viruses, bacteria and candida.

One answer to this may well be Oxytech capsules from Dulwich Health. These capsules have to be taken with plenty of water, and lots more during the day. To put it simply, when they hit your stomach, their oxygen explodes into your system, benefiting your good bacteria and creating the right environment to eliminate all the bad stuff. They are recommended for quickly getting rid of colds and flu. On a high dose, you may experience diarrhoea, but the benefits outweigh the temporary nuisance. The other snag is, they are very expensive. Full details of this treatment are available from Dulwich Health (see page 182).

Physiotherapy

This treatment should provide M.E. sufferers with some good alternatives to drugs for some common problems. Physiotherapy could be particularly important if you started your M.E. with a physical injury.

Physiotherapists may be able to help M.E. sufferers in a number of ways, giving advice on exercise, lifestyle and pain relief.

Exercises

We read a lot about graduated exercise programmes, about which I am very dubious. I consider paced 'graduated pottering' the best sort of exercise, and even then there will be some days when it might be wiser to stop.

However, when you are a lot better and feel up to it, a physiotherapist could give you some very gentle, toning exercises. Severe sufferers of M.E. could find themselves literally lying down all day, hardly moving a limb. This is not desirable and it could help if a physiotherapist could visit and give very gentle passive exercises to the sufferer lying in bed. These should be within the limits of comfortable movement and not cause stress.

Hydrotherapy (exercise in water) is very helpful in maintaining strength and mobility and the warmth of the water may help ease the pain. I don't know anyone with M.E. who has tried it but I do, however, know someone who has installed a jacuzzi fitting in her bath and feels the benefit on her stiff joints early in the morning.

Some M.E. sufferers hyperventilate: professional advice on breathing exercises can be very helpful.

Relaxation

M.E. sufferers are naturally very worried about their condition and this in itself brings tension and stress. Learning to relax helps you unwind and is also beneficial in conserving and refreshing energy.

Physiotherapists can advise you on this important subject. Don't expect miracles at first. M.E. sufferers' bodies do tend to stress easily. I personally believe that relaxation techniques and tapes are very helpful, and the more you practise, the greater the benefits will be.

Pain relief

Physiotherapists use a number of methods to relieve pain. These include acupuncture, electrotherapy, exercises, hydrotherapy, manual therapy, massage and advice on pain control, e.g. posture and how to get the best out of your hot water bottle!

Physiotherapy can be obtained both on the NHS and in private clinics. Unfortunately, most NHS physiotherapy departments are overloaded and a service for M.E. sufferers is not universally available, but it is worth enquiring.

Reflexology

This ancient art of healing goes back thousands of years to the early Egyptians and Chinese. It helps the body relax, rebalance and heal itself. According to reflexologists, every part of you is connected, by an energy pathway, to your feet. Perhaps you can imagine a mini-map of your body on the soles of your feet, split up into small areas representing all parts and organs of your body.

The reflexologist applies massage techniques and gentle pressure to all the relevant areas and can actually feel the problem zones, which we wouldn't notice. When the therapist feels a trouble spot (it will feel tender on your foot, almost like a bruise) you might possibly feel a corresponding twinge in the part of your body that has been giving you trouble although this will not necessarily be the case.

Reflexology releases tension in the feet, which in

turn eliminates toxins and improves circulation, helping your energy flow freely and correctly again. You will probably recognise similarities with treatment by acupuncture as that stimulates the same energy pathways or meridians.

Don't expect reflexology to provide an instant cure: nothing short of a miracle can do that. I think of it as an on-going boost to my immune system and an aid to pain relief. I also hope it might prevent other potential problems surfacing.

Some people think it might tickle, but it doesn't. It is a very pleasurable and relaxing therapy with no bad side effects. Some people may feel slightly worse at first, while others feel an improvement very quickly. With M.E., any improvement is likely to be slow, but anything which can help long-term or give a little boost on a particular day is worth trying.

Mental relaxation

We all know how important it is to rest the body, but the mind gets tired and stressed too. This wastes a lot of energy and is not conducive to healing. It is now recognised that relaxation and visualisation can be very helpful. Positive thoughts of when you were fit and healthy, winning a sports event at school, or even mental pictures of your immune system lining up your bad viruses for the firing squad can all be helpful! You may laugh, but try it.

Most of us, prior to suffering from M.E., would have considered sitting watching the television, reading, talking, sewing, etc. as comparatively relaxing pastimes! Now, however, you will need to 'switch off' *completely* from time to time and give those busy brains a complete rest. Watching the television actually takes far more mental energy than you would imagine, but listening to something relaxing, like gentle music, relieves you from having to think, and takes a lot less.

Relaxation is also beneficial for your thymus gland, which lies a little below your collar bones, beneath your breastbone, at the top end of your chest. To explain this simply, your thymus is the barracks where the fighting soldiers of your immune system live, ready to fend off viruses and bacteria. Strangely enough, just giving it the odd thump now and again can also revitalise it.

It is a matter of personal preference whether you listen to relaxation tapes, gentle music, visualisation tapes which take you off into another world, or the kind that explain how to relax your body bit by bit, muscle by muscle, at the end of which you may even drop off to sleep! Some tapes offer Autogenic Training (AT for short). They may help make you aware of where you hold tensions in your body, which may have gone unnoticed until now. You will need a quiet room without distractions and your eyes shut, or perhaps a Walkman, which shuts out all other noises – even the doorbell! You can also use your own imagination to conjure up pictures of pleasant surroundings, like pretty countryside or a tropical island, if you are able to. I have found mental images more difficult since having M.E., but some days are better than others.

When you feel well enough to take on a slightly more active therapy, gentle remedial yoga and meditation are known to be beneficial, but be careful not to rush into anything which will make you physically tired.

CHAPTER 6

Food and Diet

Diet is one of the most important aspects of M.E. To a large extent, we are what we eat, and when the immune system is low, what we eat is even more important. Every mouthful must be nourishing and junk food must be a thing of the past!

If you have candida and allergy problems, you may find it useful to buy specialised recipe books, often available at health food shops and book shops. Recipes are sometimes given in the free magazines from health shops too. If you cannot tolerate wheat, dairy products, yeast or sugar, you may find a book to suit your needs and there are several cookery books which deal with the anti-candida diet. However, if you have multiple allergies, these books are not so useful, as every recipe may have something in it that you can't eat. In this case, it is easier to prepare simple meals rather than complicated recipes unless you have someone to cook for you! In due course, you will find you become a master of substitution and can often eat meals you first thought impossible.

In order to build yourself up, it is essential to eat a very healthy, nutritious diet. Do not eat junk food, cakes, biscuits, sweets, fizzy drinks, or processed and convenience foods which are full of additives and E numbers. Keep salt, fatty and fried foods to the minimum and eat fresh produce wherever possible. I find tinned fish comes in handy for snack lunches and the edible bones are good to top up my calcium, but other tinned foods are best left on the shelf. I have now stopped eating sardines as I feel they contain too much mercury. Tinned fruit and vegetables are yeasty and unsuitable. Refined starch (like white bread, white rice, white pizza bases, etc.), sugary food, tea, coffee and booze are not going to improve your health. Aim for fresh meat, mostly poultry or game, fish, eggs, seafood, wholegrains, brown rice, pulses, small amounts of dairy produce (yoghurt if you can tolerate it) and stacks of fresh, steamed vegetables, fresh fruit (as permitted by your candida diet) and some raw salad. Drink plenty of bottled or filtered water. Stir-fry vegetables to retain the goodness. I always feel that although wholegrains may contain the most nutritional value, they may also contain the most pesticides and so I would advise organic bread, if possible. It can be sliced and frozen like other breads, and eaten as required to minimise waste.

If you have irritable bowel, candida or allergies, you will have to adapt your diet to suit your needs. Eat as varied a diet as possible within your own limitations, but bear in mind that many M.E. sufferers have trouble digesting fats.

Please note that protein is absolutely essential in order to make energy. You probably need at least 225 g (8 oz) to give you enough ingredients from which to manufacture your energy. On my Hay Diet, I tend to make my breakfast (the most difficult meal of the day) a starchy one, and then I eat two protein-based meals with heaps of vegetables or salad, and what limited fruits I dare between meals. This works for me, my appetite and my allergies. Work out the best system you can to suit yourself. Some people need protein early in the day to 'stoke up their boiler' and they also digest it better than later in the evening. I am probably one of the latter kind, and although limited by the Hay Diet and my allergies, I do tend to nibble protein snacks between meals to keep me going. Incidentally, raw foods like fruit, salad and carrots are good for us because they haven't had all the goodness cooked out of them. Organic or garden vegetables are the safest choice. Try to eat plenty (before a meal is a good time), but not so much that it upsets your tummy!

Although I have never read any particular warnings for M.E. sufferers with regard to food poisoning, anyone with a weak immune system should take extra care with their diet. It is sensible to follow the government advice issued to pregnant women, babies and the elderly on the following:

- **Chicken:** cook right through. Leftover chicken inadequately reheated can be extremely dangerous.

- **Eggs:** cook through and avoid raw ones (beware of home-made mayonnaise).

- **Soft cheeses:** those made from unpasteurised milk are better avoided.

Tips for difficult diets

For anyone who has been able to eat just about anything, including ready-prepared or junk food, going on any sort of new diet is going to be difficult at first. The first rule is fresh, nutritious ingredients, freshly prepared as often as possible. Generally speaking, the more we chop, slice, soak, store, boil, freeze and reheat our food, the less goodness it will have left in it. I find reheated lamb, as in shepherd's pie, very indigestible. For people who suddenly become sensitive to food substances, diet can become even more difficult. It may help if you write down in advance a list of what you can eat and easily prepare, rather than relying on a foggy brain to try and think of something for lunch at the last minute. If you keep a diary, it will help you see which foods are upsetting you.

The biggest problem is knowing whether to eat foods we are sensitive to or not. Opinions vary a bit on this! If we eat 'sensitive' food, this may use up valuable energy that could be put to better use, and can also give us unpleasant symptoms. If we religiously avoid everything that might be upsetting us, this will narrow the diet greatly and deprive us of many vitamins and minerals. I try to take the middle road but I do avoid all foods that do me more harm than good. You will soon discover what you can safely get away with! Eat as wide a variety of food as possible. You may be able to reintroduce sensitive foods later on.

The Hay Diet

Most people have heard of this diet but not everyone knows what it involves. It is a very healthy eating pattern for life. The main basic principle is the separation of proteins and starches at the same meal. This is easier on the digestive system and allows you to get the most out of your food. This means no more fish and chips, steak pie or meat curry with rice. However, it is not a depriving diet as all good food can be eaten, as long as it is correctly combined with other food at the same meal.

It would seem that very healthy people can get away with eating what they like (for a while anyway) but ill people really benefit from taking extra care of their digestive systems. M.E. sufferers often have digestive problems, such as irritable bowel and indigestion, plus allergies and weight problems. Long-term, the Hay Diet could help with these and more besides; in fact, everyone who tries it says that they notice a difference with their digestive system immediately. Over the last two years, it has also greatly relieved my urticaria (itchy skin rashes which drove me mad).

If, like me, you have many allergies and candida which already affect your diet, you will find you cannot follow the Hay Diet in every last detail, but the diet can be adapted to suit your individual requirements and the correct combining of foods can be followed quite easily.

The Hay Diet is often promoted as a diet for weight reduction, but it is really a balancing diet. If you are too thin, it could help you put a bit of weight on as you will digest your food better. If you are too heavy, its sensible combination of lots of vegetables with less starch could help you slowly lose weight. It does involve one unusual rule: don't drink at meal times. I found this difficult as I take pills around meal times. I have read a conflicting view, which suggests that it doesn't matter when you drink as long as you drink water. No one drinks enough water, it seems. Anyway, as long as you separate starch from protein, you will probably feel the benefit. If you do drink at meal times, don't use the water to swill down large lumps of food – chew it well! Digestion of carbohydrates actually starts in the mouth.

Diet tips for candida sufferers

If you have candida, make sure everything you eat is very fresh. Leftovers in the fridge start to grow 'invisible' moulds. Plenty of fibre will be needed to 'blot up' the toxins and lots of water to swill them through. Avoid heavy fatty foods and red meat, but concentrate on chicken, turkey, game, fish and seafood, perhaps with a little liver. Lamb would appear to be slightly more naturally reared than beef and pork, though non-organic lamb has, of course, been soaked to the skin with sheep dip (dangerous organo-phosphates).

Salad and vegetables are good to eat, with the exception of mushrooms (and truffles!). Fruit juices are too high in concentrated fruit sugar and fruit needs to be limited, especially at first, for the same reason. I find I can eat acidic fruit like apples, berries and pineapple (all fresh). Avoid sweet fruits like bananas, grapes, melons, figs and very juicy, ripe pears.

Eggs are fine if you can tolerate them. Any grains you are not allergic to must be whole, wherever possible. Brown rice is probably better for the digestive system than wheat. I recommend that you take care with dairy products, but if you are intolerant of them, as many of us are, you won't be greatly tempted by them anyway.

Yeasts love eating sugar and thrive on it. Diets high in sugar and refined, starchy food will make the condition worse. Fermented substances like alcohol and vinegar need to be avoided too. Most candida sufferers are intolerant of yeast, which is present in many foods.

Some experts say that dairy products create a bad environment for the bowel and should be avoided. They may also be responsible for a lot of joint pain. In any case, cheese (especially the smelly, mouldy ones) should be avoided altogether, and probably milk as it contains milk sugar (lactose). I thoroughly enjoyed soya milk, until I had too much of it and couldn't take it at all. Be warned! Some people can manage a tiny bit of butter, which is probably better for us than most margarine anyway, and some can manage a *little* natural live yoghurt, if they think it is a good idea. The choice is yours!

Fresh food is recommended, rather than pre-packed foods. The diet can be improved by cooking your own soups, pâtés and stocks, if you have someone to help! If food has suddenly become a bit bland, use fresh herbs to liven it up.

It is a good idea to wash all fruits and vegetables thoroughly to get rid of as much invisible mould as possible. A solution of potassium permanganate will remove all the 'hidden nasties' on fruit and vegetables. Dissolve two grains in a pint of water, soak fruit and vegetables for ten minutes, rinse and eat. Some doctors advise peeling apples and pears, as they may be waxed to give them a sheen and this grease doesn't seem to wash off. Incidentally, it is better to eat fruits between meals: up to 15 minutes *before* a meal is all right, but not *after* food. This may seem a bit back-to-front, but the reason is that a protein or starch meal will take a long time to digest and will cause a 'traffic jam', leaving the fruit to ferment in the queue.

One man's meat is another man's poison they say, and so it is for candida sufferers. Here is a list of foods you should avoid:

- Sugar – described in Leon Chaitow's book *Candida Albicans* as 'Pure, white and deadly' – and any sugar-containing foods. Read all food labels carefully. Sugar is often hidden in foods like ice cream, baked beans, sauces and cereals and comes in the guise of sucrose, dextrose, maltose, lactose, fructose, sorbitol and corn syrup. Even the so-called healthy sugars like molasses, maple syrup and honey are definitely out! Particularly watch out for sorbitol, which is known to badly upset people's tummies. You can even buy sugar-free natural toothpaste from health shops.

122

- Any food containing yeast: bread, buns, Oxo cubes, Bisto, Marmite, Bovril, spreads, etc.

- Food supplements containing yeast.

- Anything fermented: alcohol obviously, but also vinegar and soy sauce. Miso, Quorn, tempeh, tofu, which are used a lot by vegetarians, are also fermented and not suitable.

- Anything malted: Ovaltine, malt bread, cereals and even bean sprouts.

- Foods high in moulds: dried fruit, spices. Mushrooms (and truffles), which are actually edible mould.

- Pickles, sauces, mayonnaise, mint sauce and most bottles of tasty stuff!

- Drinks high in fruit sugar (fructose), such as squashes, cordials and fizzy drinks. Home-made juices, e.g. vegetable juices, are fine.

- Canned and frozen fruit drinks and citric acid in any drinks.

- Tea, coffee, cola and chocolate (sorry!). You could try herbal teas, Rooibosch tea and dandelion or chicory coffee, but they are unsuitable for some. Rice Dream is a good new drink made from organic brown rice, safflower oil, filtered water and sea salt, which should be safe for many. Green tea is healthy, but does contain some caffeine.

- Red meats: beef, in particular, is often an allergy problem.

- Refined starch in any form as it turns easily to sugar inside you. Whole grains are more appropriate and nutritious. Rice, millet, corn and oats will probably be better than wheat for most people.

- Some doctors advise *no* sticky, gluten-containing grains, i.e. wheat, oats, barley and rye.

- Food covered in crumbs (this will mostly be frozen!).

- Additives, preservatives, flavourings and colourings, especially monosodium glutamate, which is very yeasty.

- Nuts, unless very fresh, preferably just shelled. Peanuts should never be eaten – they are very mouldy and many people are allergic to them. Avoid peanut butter too.

- Dairy products, including fromage frais, crème fraîche, sour cream and buttermilk, with the possible exception of a little butter and natural live yoghurt, if tolerated. Cheese and milk are the worst offenders.

- Smoked meats often contain yeast and additives. An occasional treat of smoked haddock or kipper should be naturally smoked and pale in colour.

- Artificial sweeteners are often synthetic

chemicals. I am sensitive to them (aspartame gave me cystitis) and so I wouldn't touch them anyway.

- As you have probably guessed by now, water is the best, and sometimes the only, drink. Have plenty, preferably filtered or bottled.

If this is a bit much to take in at first, remember there is still plenty of good, healthy stuff to eat. We are all human, I know, and we all think about cheating (especially if no one is watching!). However, if we eat something that upsets us, we suffer for it and are only cheating ourselves. If you just know that you must eat something sinful or burst, a square or two of carob-type chocolate will be better than half a bar of real, sugary chocolate, even though carob is not actually recommended!

In spite of some people's remarks about our 'lunatic diets', I consider this to be a very healthy diet as it excludes a lot of harmful junk food. For me it would be lunatic to eat what I fancy, as that would keep me permanently ill.

Breakfasts

Breakfast is usually the most difficult meal for the sensitive, so I will give a few suggestions which may help, depending on your allergies.

Oats, as in muesli or porridge	Do not eat if you have a problem with all gluten-containing cereals. Porridge can be made with water – as a last resort!

125

Millet flakes with soya milk	Also make a very quick porridge with milk or water
Roasted buckwheat (no relation of wheat) and quinoa	Available in health food shops
Sugar-free rice crispies or cornflakes	Helpful for many, if you can manage a little milk, soya milk or juice to moisten. I have eaten them dry, but it is difficult
Potato dishes, such as bubble and squeak	Some people are allergic to the potato family of foods, which includes aubergines, tomatoes and peppers
Sweet potato, sautéed with onion, garlic, herbs, etc.	Helps to add variety
Rice cakes and corn	Various varieties available from health shops and some supermarkets
Natural live yoghurt with linseeds	Some people can manage a very little yoghurt though allergic to dairy produce in general. I eat sheep's yoghurt

Fruit	Eat only small amounts if you suffer from candida
Buckwheat and maizemeal pancakes, with a smear of sugar-free jam, or better still, olive pâté	Can be made with water and egg instead of milk, or even without egg – keep the mixture thick and pancakes small, or they will tend to fall to bits
Gluten-free sausages	Delicious and filling if you can get them. May still contain monosodium glutamate and additives
Smoked haddock or kippers	Don't eat smoked food very often

If even these breakfasts upset you, you may have to resort to 'non-breakfast' food, for example, home-made pâté, soup, rice and pulses or vegetables, or even a good salad.

For those of you who can drink little more than water, here are a few more suggestions for drinks to start your day.

- Infuse fresh herbs, rosemary, apple mint, ginger mint, etc. in hot water. Root ginger is warming too.

- Make juices with carrot, tomato, cabbage, beet-root and apple combinations. Do not, however, drink gallons of carrot juice as you may turn bright orange and expire of vitamin A poisoning!

Meat and sausages

There are various companies selling organic meat direct to the customer, as well as through selected butchers. Containing no antibiotics or artificial hormones, this is much safer to eat. It can be delivered to your home in bulk (probably 12 lbs minimum) and, with the delivery charge, would mean spending about £50 at one time which inevitably means freezing. It is difficult to assess how much goodness is lost by freezing meat. It has been suggested to me that as the frozen juices thaw, when defrosting, some nutrients will leach out.

If you happen to live near an organic butcher, you may be able to pick up a little organic meat when required and eat it fresh. It is more expensive but is supposed to taste better. I made enquiries, from the Real Meat company mentioned at the back of the book, about sodium nitrite and nitrate in organic bacon. It seems that they are an integral part of bacon, even though the pork started out as organic.

More recently, I have tried meat from a company at Swaddles Green Farm, which I found to be dense and filling and therefore actually more economical than it first seems. You can order as much or as little as you need.

Some butchers might make you a batch of gluten-free sausages, if you ask nicely. However, the ones I bought still contained monosodium glutamate and preservatives, which upset me.

'Simply Sausages' in London (see page 184) make a

large range of beautiful sausages, some gluten-free, some vegetarian, with natural skins and no additives or preservatives. They specialise in sausages which are good and solid enough for breakfast, lunch or supper. If you have a kind friend or neighbour who works in London, perhaps they would get you some. This shouldn't be a problem when they get hooked on them themselves! This is something I do freeze as I buy them in bulk. They wouldn't keep long in the fridge due to the lack of preservatives.

Butter or margarine

Many experts now accept that natural butter is healthier than margarine, as the hydrogenation process margarine has to go through, to turn it from a liquid into something spreadable, involves mixing it with nickel and heating it more than once to very high temperatures, neither of which is healthy or desirable. For those allergic to butter, Vitaquell (available from health food shops) may be a suitable alternative. It is a healthy spread, unhydrogenated, and you can cook with it. Vitaquell contains maize and wheatgerm oils, but Vitaquell Cuisine (for cooking) does not specify which oils it contains. I get on well with it, but also use small amounts of cold-pressed olive oil for pan cooking. Whole Earth is another quality unhydrogenated soft spread made from soya beans. I am pleased to see there is now a tendency for more conventional margarines to be unhydrogenated.

Cooking oils

The best oils for cooking or salads are the natural ones that have not been refined, heated and processed; that means cold-pressed olive oil and unrefined oils, such as safflower or sunflower. Cold-pressed olive oil is a good salad dressing, especially for candida sufferers. It is also the most stable oil for cooking. Never heat oils to smoking and make sure you use it only once.

Water

Water comes from springs, boreholes, reservoirs and lakes, picking up pollution and mineral content according to its location. It is therefore thought to be safer to drink bottled or filtered water than tap water. Over the years, there have been scares with excessive levels of aluminium, chemicals and even pesticides in our water. Even fluoride may not be the 'goodie' it was made out to be. Lead from pipes is toxic, nitrates can be too high, and apart from anything else, the chlorine tastes nasty! However, even bottled water is not perfect as it may contain high levels of bacteria. Good-quality Scottish water in glass bottles is probably best, as plastic contains nasty chemicals and some people are highly allergic to plastic.

Apparently good spring water is better than mineral water unless the body is deficient in those minerals. Excessive intake of minerals can lead to problems with our delicate water balance. The purer the water, the better it is for our bodies. As in a car battery, minerals clog the electrolytic system, the basic energy of life. Drinking a lot of mineral water could induce kidney stones, so I put mine through a jug filter as well. It doesn't get everything out, but it helps. Mineral water does have the advantage of being regulated, whereas spring water does not. Malvern, Buxton, Evian, Highland Spring and Volvic are said to be the best that are readily available.

If you drink bottled water, please observe the drink-by date. Once opened, water should be consumed in a day or two at room temperature, or within a week if kept in the refrigerator.

An efficient domestic water filter, or a water filter jug, is an economical alternative. Make sure you change the filter frequently and give it a regular clean out as per the instructions.

You may wish to consider having a filter plumbed into your water supply. These systems can cost over £500, however, and there are arguments both for and against them. For more information, read *Food Allergy and Intolerance* by Dr Jonathan Brostoff and Linda Gamlin (see list at back of book).

Health food shops

If illness and food sensitivities are limiting what you can eat, you will find in health food shops a wide range of specialised food, which will give you a greater variety and better balanced diet. For people sensitive to cereals, sugar and dairy products, it is helpful to find suitable alternatives, such as:

- Soya milk (sugar-free if necessary), yoghurt and cheese

- Sugar-free cereals such as rice and cornflakes

- Alternative flours: buckwheat, soy, chickpea and maize

- Alternative grains such as millet, roast buckwheat and quinoa

- Rice cakes

- Healthy alternatives to butter

- Sugar-free jam

There should also be quite a lot of food suitable for vegetarians, along with a host of supplements, which can be specially ordered if necessary. Many health food shops also offer a mail-order service.

It is possible to pick up free health magazines, which include all sorts of interesting features like recipes and information on supplements, etc. You may also find an article on M.E. now and then. If you cannot get out yourself, perhaps a friend or relative could pick them up for you.

My local shop has a good selection of books on health subjects, including M.E. If you have trouble with, say, cystitis, or are wondering if royal jelly might help you, there will most likely be a helpful book on the matter.

If you do find something really useful in the food line, remember not to eat too much as you are more likely to become sensitive to it and so have to avoid it altogether! The bulk of your diet should still be fresh food.

Weight

The majority of M.E. sufferers tend to lose weight, especially in the early stages, due to nausea, lack of appetite, malabsorption, irritable bowel or simply being asleep for hours on end and only grabbing quick little nibbles. Later, those following an anti-candida diet and eliminating their sugar and refined starches will also lose a few pounds. M.E. does sometimes tend to nibble away at the muscles; also, anyone confined to a bed or a wheelchair for long periods may have extra problems due to lack of mobility and exercise.

However, some sufferers with good appetites but little mobility may actually put on weight and will need to cut down on naughty starches but still eat a very healthy diet.

Anyone worried about extreme weight gain or loss should consult a doctor in case there are thyroid or water retention problems involved.

CHAPTER 7

Supplements

This subject is a minefield where, as a sufferer and not a doctor, I hardly dare to tread. It is true that a little knowledge can be dangerous and, if at all possible, it is advisable to seek expert advice from a specialist in the field of nutrition. I have spoken to two specialists, one specialising in clinical nutrition, and have picked up some useful information. General reading has also helped. If possible, it would be a good start to have some specific blood tests to see what you are deficient in, but without private health insurance, this may be very expensive.

Many people think that as long as we eat a healthy diet, we should not need supplements. In reality, we can easily be deficient in various vitamins and minerals and it is most unlikely that an M.E. sufferer would not be deficient in something. M.E. specialists recognise that illness, stress, candida, allergies, etc. deplete our resources quickly. The majority of M.E. sufferers have digestive troubles and many may not be absorbing their nourishment properly, in spite of a good diet. Most sufferers resort to supplements as part of their management plan and most doctors encourage it. Always remember, however, that supplements are not meant to replace good food: a nutritious diet is the first essential and is more easily absorbed than pills. Supplements are there to fill the gaps caused by malabsorption and restrictive diets;

however, anyone with a leaky gut or suffering from geopathic stress will not get the full benefit from dietary supplements.

Specialist advice is the ideal but, if you have to do it by yourself, perhaps I can offer some guidance. It is no good going into a health food shop and picking up a selection at random. Vitamins and minerals rely on one another to do their job properly. They work together as a team and if one of the team doesn't turn up, they don't perform properly (just as a football team wouldn't perform well without a goalie).

A good multi-vitamin and mineral supplement would ensure that you got a bit of everything, then you could add to it as your needs require. However, just because a certain supplement may be good for you, it doesn't mean that heaps of it will be even better. On the contrary, overdosing can be dangerous, particularly with vitamins A and D.

Most supplements are taken with food: always read the label for instructions. Oils are supposed to be more effective between meals but can be taken with food if your digestive system is delicate. If you react badly to a supplement, stop taking it. And do remember: too much of a good thing can give toxic symptoms and *anybody* can be sensitive to *anything*, even natural herbal substances.

The following pages provide a list of vitamins and minerals which could be of benefit to you.

Vitamin B complex

This is essential for immune system function and is best taken at breakfast time. It is better to take the whole B complex than isolated items as they work better as a team. Choose a yeast-free brand.

Vitamin C

This vitamin helps fight bacterial and viral activity and is considered very important in the treatment of M.E. It needs to be taken at intervals throughout the day as the body cannot store it. The brands labelled 'buffered' are kinder to the digestive system.

Vitamin A/beta carotene

These, too, fight viral activity. Beta carotene is preferable as the body takes what it needs and turns it into vitamin A. This is a safe way of taking a potentially toxic vitamin.

Vitamin E

Vitamin E is also helpful in enhancing the effective functioning of the immune system.

Selenium

Very useful for immune system function when taken in small quantities. Find a yeast-free brand.

Zinc

Probably the single most important mineral, this one is captain of your immune system. White spots on finger nails can indicate a deficiency. Best taken at night by itself, without food.

Magnesium, calcium

Many M.E. sufferers are deficient in magnesium, which is best taken with calcium, as they work as a pair. Solgar's calcium and magnesium has added boron, which is good for the bones.

BioCare produce forms of magnesium which are readily absorbed, such as Bio-magnesium and EAP.

Multi-vitamin and multi-mineral tablets

These will include some extra items, such as kelp, chromium, potassium, iron and manganese, and complete your team.

Vitamin B$_{12}$

B$_{12}$ may sometimes be administered by injection or sub-lingually.

Buying supplements

When buying supplements, it is worth getting the best you can afford. Solgar and Blackmore are two very good brands to look for and BioCare and Lamberts are good mail order companies (see pages 182–3).

Action for M.E. produce an excellent fact sheet on vitamins and minerals. Their introductory tape for M.E. sufferers also gives very good advice on diet and explains how to manage on the minimum of supplements – this is important as the cost of good-quality supplements can be considerable and you may be on a tight budget, particularly if you have had to stop work as a result of your illness.

Members of the M.E. Association or Action for M.E. can obtain discounts on goods from several manufacturers and distributors of supplements, including BioCare and Dulwich Health.

The associations also sell evening primrose oil (see pages 144–5) cheaply to members; this product is expensive but extremely valuable, so if you can afford the initial outlay, buy the large economy size.

Literally hundreds of supplements are available; here is a list of those which I think you may find most useful.

Alfalfa

This plant's roots burrow down 30 feet, and often more, to reach valuable minerals and vitamins not available at the soil's surface. It also has anti-inflammatory properties.

Aloe vera juice

Aloe vera is extracted from the centre of a thick, fleshy leaf of a cactus-like plant in the lily family. It is a natural antibiotic and has great healing qualities. In common with royal jelly, it contains a long list of healthy ingredients, including vitamins, minerals, amino acids and enzymes. It has also been found to contain vitamin B_{12}, which is normally found only in foods high in protein, such as meat, fish, chicken, cheese, milk and eggs. This could be good news for vegetarians. Deficiency in B_{12} can cause a host of nasty symptoms, many of which are found in M.E.

(fatigue, weakness, forgetfulness, dizziness, head-aches and many more).

For candida sufferers, aloe vera juice is said to help heal a 'leaky gut'. It makes a pleasant drink between meals. Cold stabilised brands, which contain no sorbitol, are available at health shops. I use Life Stream by Xynergy Health Products.

This juice is enjoying great popularity at the moment and many M.E. sufferers have found that a concentrated three-month course has yielded great benefits. However, please note that some brands contain a very low percentage of aloe vera juice, whilst others have too much sorbitol, which badly upsets some people's tummies and may make their M.E. symptoms worse. Sorbitol is corn syrup which in itself may induce an allergic reaction.

Aloe vera must not be taken by pregnant women.

Amino acids

These are essential to good health. There are many of them, each with its own job to do. There is no way of telling if we are deficient in them, but this is quite possible if we are not digesting our protein properly. I will draw your attention to three of them, which have an important role to play in M.E.

• **Glutamic acid (glutamine):** this amino acid is known as 'brain fuel' and may also be helpful to the lining of the digestive tract. It is useful in controlling hypoglycaemia and cravings for sweet things and is recommended for people with stomach ulcers. Cabbage is a rich source of glutamic acid.

- **Tyrosine:** tyrosine, the second amino acid, helps the thyroid to function properly and may also be helpful in depression: these are both common in M.E. Your body will make its own tyrosine from another amino acid called phenylalanine, which may help with pain relief. However, never take it in large quantities, such as in a single supplement, if you suffer from severe depression: it can produce unpleasant side effects.

- **Lysine:** lysine has anti-viral properties, particularly against herpes viruses, such as chicken pox and glandular fever, which sometimes trigger M.E. Lysine damps down the virus's enthusiasm to multiply. From lysine, our body manufactures carnitine, which has a role to play in the manufacture of energy.

Amino acids can be obtained from Solgar and mail order companies. It is recommended that amino acids be taken between meals. It is also wise to take them as a complex rather than individually. Syner Protein nutritional drink, made by Nature's Sunshine, is an excellent example, although it is not always well tolerated by people suffering from M.E.

Lysine-rich food can also help in the battle against the virus, whilst too much food rich in arginine (another amino acid) will be unhelpful. Leon Chaitow's book *Postviral Fatigue Syndrome* explains this and gives lists of suitable and unsuitable foods. Ensuring optimum levels of amino acids is quite a complicated subject and expert advice is advisable. Never take any long-term without a break.

Bioflavenoids

These are the natural colourings in soft fruits such as bilberries, blackcurrants, raspberries and cranberries.

It is thought that by strengthening the blood-brain barrier they may help in preventing brain lesions which occur in M.E. sufferers. Unfortunately, tests have not yet established what the correct dose should be.

Lamberts produce capsules called Colladeen, which contain extracts of cranberry, bilberry, grape seed and pine bark. They contain anti-inflammatory and anti-oxidant properties. They are NOT suitable for pregnant women.

Butyric acid

Our bodies produce this in the bowel and it is also found in butter and olive oil. The production of this acid can be helped by eating fibre and pulses. Like aloe vera, it will help heal a leaky gut (caused by candida), is mildly antifungal, may help some acidophilus supplements to 'stick' where they belong, and is also supposed to be beneficial in alleviating food allergies. It is available in supplement form from BioCare, but I reacted to this particular supplement with a headache, so I always use olive oil as a salad dressing to boost my intake.

Cat's claw

This herb from the Peruvian rain forest comes from a vine with large thorns resembling cats' claws. It has antiviral and anti-inflammatory properties and is said to be helpful to the digestive system. It claims the ability to strengthen the immune system and may help people with M.E., candida and depression. It should not be taken during pregnancy.

Chlorella

Chlorella is similar to spirulina and blue-green algae. It is at the start of the freshwater food chain and full of nourishment. It contains over 20 vitamins and minerals, including iron and B_{12}; this is good news for everyone, especially vegetarians. It assists the growth of tissue and repairs damage; it is an immune system booster; it helps detoxify our bodies, even binding with lead, mercury and cadmium and helping to eliminate them. Seaweed, eaten as food, also has this ability.

Coenzyme Q10 (COQ10)

This supplement helps convert food into energy and may be useful for some people. It was discovered over 30 years ago as a natural ingredient essential to life. Your liver converts coenzyme Q10 into Q10 which gives the energy to your cells to operate your heart, muscles and liver. Unfortunately, if you are ill, your liver does not convert enough Q10. Most pharmacists as well as health shops stock Q10 but make sure you buy Q10 in soya oil (brown capsules) for the best absorption. Super Bio-Quinone Q10 is highly recommended. The normal dose is one 30mg capsule a day, but very ill people may need up to four.

143

It is said to be a very safe supplement, but as ever, check with your doctor or a clinical nutritionist.

Digestive enzymes

These are substances which our bodies produce to break down and digest our food. They may not function so well during illness or with advancing years and may be purchased as supplements at health food shops or through mail order to help the digestive system. They are often recommended for problems of candida, allergies, malabsorption and general digestive troubles, recognised by bloating, irritable bowel, allergy and indigestion, headaches and even skin problems.

Don't expect pills to do everything for you, though. You should always chew food well, especially starch; eat good-quality food with plenty of fibre, and sufficient protein for energy; drink plenty of liquid, especially water. Digestion works best when you are relaxed, and very hot or very cold things, like tea and ice cream, are not helpful.

It is said that supplements of vegetable origin are more effective than those of animal origin, and therefore, of course, acceptable to vegetarians.

Many fruits and vegetables naturally contain high levels of digestive enzymes. These are cabbages, mangoes, carrots, bananas, tomatoes, oranges, cucumbers, grapefruit, endives, lemons, avocados, pawpaws, pineapples and fresh figs.

Echinacea

Greatly boosts the immune system against bacterial and viral infection.

Eleutherococcus senticosus (ES, or Siberian ginseng)

This herb is often confused with ginseng and does have some similarities. They both help the body adapt to difficult circumstances. ES has the greater healing powers without the possible side effects of ginseng. Although it is not a stimulant, it increases strength, endurance and concentration. For these reasons, it has in the past been found helpful for athletes, invalids in convalescence and anyone taking exams. Some M.E. sufferers are now finding it beneficial in treating their energy, joint pain and brain problems.

It is considered to be very safe unless you have high blood pressure, when expert advice and careful monitoring are essential. However safe herbs are considered to be, it would be unwise to go on dosing oneself indefinitely without professional advice.

Evening primrose oil

Primrose oil is good for so many different things: hair, skin, nails, eczema, pre-menstrual tension, allergies, arthritis, multiple sclerosis and more. It has helped to alleviate some sufferers' fatigue, muscle pain, dizziness, palpitations, mental fogginess and depression. To be of any use though, it is thought necessary to take eight capsules each day in four lots of two for at least three months. You can build up this dose gradually and, if you find it beneficial, continue and after a while perhaps reduce the dose gradually, reviewing the situation from time to time. This supplement works best if helped by certain vitamins and minerals. In Efamol, it is already combined with vitamin E for maximum efficiency, but it would probably be helpful to take a good quality multi-mineral and vitamin supplement too.

Efamol is quite safe for most people as it is a natural product, but anyone suffering from epilepsy or schizophrenia should seek medical advice before taking it.

If it should give rise to indigestion, take primrose oil with food; otherwise between meals is considered to be best.

Efamol Marine is a mixture of primrose oil and marine fish oil and clinical trials have proven it can be of real benefit to M.E. sufferers. In spite of a good diet, many people cannot manufacture and extract from their food this most important essential fatty acid, called GLA for short. It is responsible for many aspects of health and is particularly relevant to the brain, central nervous system, blood and resistance to infection.

Our bodies cannot make GLA naturally and so we rely on certain foods for it: dairy products, liver, kidneys and vegetable seed oils, such as unrefined sunflower or safflower oils. It is also found in human breast milk. Unfortunately, many people are allergic to dairy products, don't like offal, use the wrong sort of cooking oils and, let's face it, there's not much breast milk at Tesco's at the moment!

Even if we eat a lot of these products, we cannot necessarily convert them into GLA for many reasons, such as zinc deficiency, ageing, stress, alcohol, allergies, fatty foods, too much sugar, and (very relevant to M.E.) viral infections. Don't worry though: in Efamol Marine, you have the complete 'do-it-yourself' package.

Ginger

Ginger is a useful spice, which can be used for purposes other than gingerbread and biscuits. It is very warming and aids circulation. It assists digestion and many people find that it helps to relieve nausea and vomiting.

I have made drinks with root ginger and hot water and also taken it in supplement form. M.E. sufferers do take a bit of warming up, but I found that a warm bath, a ginger drink and a hot water bottle did have a good effect on me, even if it was only temporary.

Ginkgo biloba

This is a natural product, derived from the ginkgo biloba tree, which may help poor circulation. Some M.E. sufferers have found it useful for memory, concentration and cold feet. However, is is not suitable for anyone with a heart problem.

Golden seal

This herb has a soothing effect on internal passages. It is a powerful herb with a natural antibiotic effect and it would be prudent to consult a herbalist before taking it. Do not take it if you are pregnant.

Hydrochloric acid

Some M.E. sufferers have been found to be low in stomach acid, needed to digest their food. This can be boosted with a supplement of hydrochloric acid. However, don't take hydrochloric acid supplements if you have any sort of internal ulcers. This is strong stuff and it would be wise to seek medical advice and be tested first.

Iodine

DO NOT take iodine by mouth. It can be safely and effectively absorbed through the skin, either by rubbing on the inner thighs (using cotton wool and rubber gloves) or by soaking your feet in a bowl of water containing 10 drops of iodine. I have found that 15 minutes is enough for my body to absorb all it needs.

Treat iodine with care: too much can be dangerous and may cause malfunction of the thyroid. VEGA testing will tell you if you are deficient in iodine and require a supplement.

Liquorice root

Liquorice root enhances the immune system and helps the function of the adrenal glands; it is also good for stress. However, it shouldn't be taken if you have high blood pressure or heart disease and, if it is taken for an extended period of time, extra potassium is recommended. This can be taken in supplement form and bananas are full of it, if you can tolerate them.

Linseeds

These can be very helpful for stomach and bowel problems. Like psyllium, they swell up when taken with liquid and help regular, gentle elimination. They can be taken in several ways, for example sprinked on cereals, yoghurt and soups, or between meals in milk or juice. The better they are chewed, the more benefit you will get out of them. They also contain essential fatty acids. I would recommend Linusit Gold.

Milk thistle

Milk thistle is said to heal and protect the liver, which in M.E. sufferers may be underfunctioning. It is available in tablet form from Solgar.

Pollen tablets

These are rich in protein and amino acids, and are recommended to help allergies. Health shops often stock Melbrosia, which combines pollen and royal jelly with vitamin C. Cernilton tablets, available from Dulwich Health, are pure pollen and provide concentrated nutrition in the form of vitamins, amino acids, trace elements and more. However, should you happen to be sensitive to a food in the same family as a pollen you consume, you may find the symptoms are triggered when you eat that particular food.

Propolis

This substance is made by the bees from collected resins from bark and buds of specific trees and plants. It is a natural antibiotic and has antiseptic qualities. To this end, it protects the hive from

149

bacterial and viral infection. It was used in ancient times for healing. It is said to have mild anaesthetic and anti-inflammatory properties and may help fight infection. For M.E. sufferers, it may be useful for the sore throat and coated tongue. It may be purchased direct from a bee-keeper or bought from a health shop under various brand names. Some M.E. sufferers have also found their energy is boosted by taking it on a regular basis and I have managed to ward off a couple of minor colds by taking good doses at the onset.

Please note that some people are allergic to propolis and other bee products. Asthmatics in particular should beware.

Royal jelly

Royal jelly contains a long list of vitamins, minerals, trace elements and amino acids. The only adverse comments I have read about royal jelly are that it can't possibly help, as the quantities involved are too small. However, it is a well-known fact that vitamins taken in the correct combinations have a far stronger effect than if taken separately.

Trials have been done with M.E. sufferers, who said that royal jelly improved their mental ability and depression. Royal jelly is also said to help with stress and strengthen the immune system.

To benefit from royal jelly, it must be taken fresh, not freeze-dried. Please note that some people are allergic to royal jelly, as with other bee products.

Salt

Too much salt is not good for us, but crystallised sea salt or organic salt, available from your health food shop, has lots of minerals and, in moderation, is essential for our bodies to function properly. If you have low blood pressure or dizziness on rising (postural hypotension) you may be low in salt and so adding a little to your diet may be helpful although it won't solve the problem completely. Muscle testing can reveal if you are low in salt. Kinesiology (see page 70) and VEGA testing (see page 73) could be useful too. Consult your doctor if you suspect your are deficient in salt. See also the sheet *Salt, Calcium and Iodine*, produced by Dulwich Health.

Tea tree oil

This natural substance comes from an Australian tree. It has been described as a complete medicine kit in a bottle as it can be used for so many purposes – up to 35 according to a leaflet in my local health shop. It is capable of killing bacteria and candida. It is able to penetrate the skin, so I use it in the bath. It should NOT be taken by mouth.

IMPORTANT:
The above list is intended solely as a guide to the benefits of supplements.

Do not take any supplements on a long-term basis without reference to a doctor or nutritionist.

A qualified medical herbalist can treat you in a holistic way, combining many herbs in one bottle.

151

CHAPTER 8

Help and Where to Find It

When you are suffering from M.E., you are at your lowest ebb. You may not have the energy to ask for help, even if you knew where to find it.

There are many organisations which can offer you assistance, from government departments to small self-help groups. In this chapter, I shall list the ones you should find most useful. The addresses and telephone numbers are at the back of the book.

Social Services

There are several social security benefits which may apply to you if you, or a member of your family, has M.E. The benefits system is rather complicated, but staff at your local Department of Social Security will help you to sort out which you can apply for. Remember, however, it is essential that you have a firm diagnosis of your condition from your doctor BEFORE you start seeking benefits.

Incapacity Benefit

This is the old Invalidity Benefit (the name was changed in April 1995) and is applicable to those who have lost their jobs through their illness and therefore have no income.

Disability Living Allowance

This combines the Attendance Allowance and Mobility Allowance. It is available to the most severely affected.

Severe Disablement Allowance

This is for people who have not been able to work for at least 28 weeks but cannot get Incapacity Benefit because they have not paid enough National Insurance contributions.

Disability Working Allowance

If you are able to work an average of 16 hours a week but your illness limits your capacity to work longer, you may be eligible to claim the disability working allowance benefit.

If you are claiming any of the above benefits, you may also be eligible for extra money for any children you may have. Your carer, if you have one, may also be able to claim an allowance.

Finding out about benefits can be an exhausting business in itself: if you cannot cope with telephone calls and filling out forms, you can get help from a social worker (ask at your doctor's surgery), or try your local Citizens' Advice Bureau – the number of your local office will be in your telephone directory or Yellow Pages.

There is also the Social Services Homecare Benefits Enquiry Line. You can talk to trained advisers on Freeline 0800 882200 between 8.30 am and 6.30 pm on weekdays or 9.00 am to 1.00 pm on Saturdays.

They will offer practical advice on things like help with form-filling and, if necessary, will send you a letter summarising the advice they have given you.

Home Help

When you need help at home, it is a good idea to get a doctor's letter before approaching Social Services. Your doctor should know your condition well and this should help you to get the assistance you need. You will also be assessed by an independent social worker or occupational therapist, at your own home if necessary. If you are not satisfied with the result, you can appeal.

There are many services available for anyone who is having difficulty coping alone. These may include shopping, laundry, cooking and sometimes cleaning, although cleaning is not a high priority when services are stretched. Help is available if you cannot bathe and dress yourself and need the district nurse to pop in, or if you are too weak to be left alone.

A booklet called *Help at Home* is available from Social Services or your local library, which simply explains exactly what is available, what it costs and how to appeal if you are not satisfied. For people on very low incomes the help is free, but some will have to pay at an hourly rate calculated according to their income. Whatever you pay, it will cover all the services you require: the charge doesn't vary with the number of services.

You can also ask Social Services (Homecare) for details of local carers.

155

Free loan of wheelchairs can be arranged through your local branch of the Red Cross or your local clinic or hospital.

Meals on Wheels

This service is manned by volunteers and is often rather stretched. It is intended for the elderly and infirm, but is also available to anyone who cannot manage at home through ill health, even if they are young. The meals are available from Monday to Friday and, at the moment, cost under £1. In emergencies, perhaps this service could fill a difficult gap in your day, even if your carer might be available in the evening to provide a dinner or light supper that is suited to your specialised needs.

While I cannot vouch for the standard of food in all areas and cannot recommend sponge pudding and custard as a nutritional remedy for M.E., I know that in my home area, at least, the current staff are very good and try to provide nourishing meals with a piece of fruit as an alternative to a pudding. The vegetables, though frozen, are steamed to keep in their maximum vitamins. If you have allergies and special dietary requirements however, this service will not be suitable for you.

If you would like to try Meals on Wheels and feel you are sufficiently disabled to qualify, the first step is to ask your doctor for a medical certificate and also the contact number for your local area. If you would like further information, contact your local Social Services.

Remember, whenever you have a problem, you can contact the M.E. Association or Action for M.E., who will always do their best to help you. You can ring the M.E. Association Advice Line on (01375) 361013 between 1.30 pm and 4.00 pm on weekdays, and after 5 pm try the Listening Ear on (01375) 642466, who will give you a current number to ring on that particular evening. If you send a stamped, addressed envelope to the M.E. Association, they will send you a comprehensive benefit information pack.

As well as social services, there are many privately-run organisations which will be able to offer you support and information.

Action for M.E.

This is an association worth joining. It offers good, practical down-to-earth reading material. For a subscription of £15, you receive quite a hefty magazine three times a year. The address and telephone number are at the back of the book.

The M.E. Association

You may find it useful to join this association too, as I did. The annual subscription costs about £15 and you will receive a quarterly magazine full of good, up-to-date information on M.E. Some articles are very practical and useful, some more technical, and there are personal stories too, which are interesting and can be encouraging.

The people running the head office work very hard and if you have any problems you need to talk about or ask about, the staff are very helpful. I have given the address and telephone numbers at the back of the book.

In cases of financial hardship, it is worth enquiring about reduced or free membership.

Both these associations can suggest names of good specialists in your area. It can be a relief to talk to people who really do understand your problems, especially if your family is still bewildered by it all.

Local support groups

When you have M.E., and are housebound most of the time, you can feel very isolated. Local support groups provide company and a welcome chance to exchange information about your illness; some groups are very enterprising and have a busy social programme. This arrangement may help sufferers and carers alike. Unfortunately, there are sometimes set-backs to this plan as many people are too ill to travel to the meeting place. Also, if a local group happens, by chance, to be full of elderly M.E. sufferers who have been ill for years and didn't benefit from early diagnosis, this atmosphere will not prove to be very uplifting and optimistic for a teenager or a parent with a young family who has been recently afflicted.

On the positive side, I have discovered through my own group that it is possible to exchange a great deal of information over the telephone and by post. I keep in touch with many people, incuding teenagers and their mothers, this way.

Action for M.E. (see page 171) can provide a list of local support groups throughout the country.

If it is impossible to meet people outside the house, I think it is helpful to have friends dropping in at convenient times for short visits so that the sufferer keeps in touch with the outside world and feels more 'normal'. Very ill people should not talk for too long as this could be tiring. I am pleased to say that I am now sufficiently recovered to start my own 'Helping Hand' Support Group. I am also pleased to say that we often have a good laugh – and you know what they say about the healing powers of laughter.

CHAPTER 9

M.E. in the Family

M.E. is no respecter of age: it can affect anyone. Although it is not common in the very young, it can occur even in pre-school-aged children and there seems to be a growing incidence amongst teenagers. This is hardly surprising, however, when you think of all the stresses that adolescence brings – and with stress, down goes the immune system, letting in all those viruses which weaken the child's body, making it more susceptible to M.E.

But how can you recognise when your child really does have M.E.? Conscientious children may plod on without complaining; the more laid-back and relaxed may complain of vague symptoms which you, the parent, may put down to fussing for attention or just plain laziness. Tummy aches and headaches could be nerves at the prospect of a new school – or they could be M.E. But how can you know?

The simple answer, I'm afraid, is that you can't know for sure. But if your child is persistently tired, emotional and generally off-colour for more than a week or two, something must be wrong. You know your child better than anyone and, if you think that there is something not quite right, you are probably correct. A visit to the doctor will not do any harm – if it is M.E., the sooner you do something about it the better and if there is nothing wrong, you can breathe a hearty sigh of relief.

So how *do* you look after a child with M.E.? The answer is, of course, it will vary from one child to another. One thing however, is certain: a lot of rest is needed both at the onset of the illness and during relapses to ensure gradual recovery. Doing too much will prolong the illness. However, going to bed, doing nothing and staying there will encourage the muscles to weaken and the brain to atrophy even further. Somehow, you have to find the balance of the right amount of rest and the right amount of mental and physical stimulation.

If it is physically impossible to attempt very much, you must at least try to keep your child's mind stimulated and happy. Sound is the least taxing pastime, so favourite music and relaxation tapes are a good idea. It would be wonderful if friends would make tapes of all their bits of news if unable to visit, then the ill child could play them when in the mood, a bit at a time.

TV, tapes and videos all have their place, but I wouldn't recommend watching all day. It is very tiring and causes eye strain. Horror videos may disturb sleep and cause nightmares but funny ones would be great, as laughter really is the best natural medicine.

Sometimes pets can be a great comfort, provided allergy is not a problem.

Think of new passive hobbies like bird-watching,

photography, drawing and painting, model-making, jigsaw puzzles, etc. Sewing and knitting may be too stressful on the shoulders and eyes.

Visits from friends should be encouraged to prevent children from feeling completely cut off but do keep them short, especially in the early stages.

One 16-year-old boy I know, who is now completely better, found mental stagnation and boredom the worst enemies. His insatiable desire to read and learn kept him sane. Radio programmes and Open University kept him well informed and interested. I seem to remember that during long periods of sleep reversal, he used to read and even compute in the night! Some sufferers would have too much trouble with jazzy vision and headaches to manage this, of course.

I am aware that some cases are very bad and children may not be well enough to do anything for a while. Motivation may well be lacking and you just need to do what you can manage on a given day and rest when you need to. One mother I spoke to felt that nothing motivated a really poorly child. She said that you just have to wait until they feel a bit better and then they motivate themselves. On the brighter side, young people do have greater potential energy and regenerative powers than us 'oldies' and stand a far better chance of full recovery.

Long-term illness does inevitably mean being cooped up for long periods, so it is nice if bedrooms, dens and lounges are pleasant places to be in. Redecorating and revamping a child's bedroom may be really appreciated. Sitting by a sunny window in a comfortable chair is the next best thing to going out.

School

When children have made sufficient recovery to attempt a gradual return to normal school life, the understanding and attitude of all school staff and helpers will be crucial. Fellow pupils will also benefit from a friendly chat about this confusing subject. They find it difficult to understand how a friend can be at school one day and not the next. Also, it is worth bearing in mind that M.E. sufferers always feel worse than they look! Whatever you do, do not send a child with M.E. back to school full-time. A full school day may be too much. Start with an hour or two in the morning and build up gradually from there.

When children return to school there are many new problems ahead of them. They are no longer in the sheltered environment of the home with food, bed and bathroom to hand. There will be physical problems like stairs, and mental obstacles like set times for doing everything. Flexibility on the part of the school will make all the difference to the ill student. I wonder how many strong staff members might volunteer to carry a young child up three flights of stairs! Certainly a good friend would be appreciated for helping to carry weighty bags.

There will be problems in class too. M.E. sufferers cannot help being slow to grasp new concepts. Their memory and concentration have suffered and they may have visual problems and uncontrolled handwriting. (I still can't read half my shopping lists!) If the lesson becomes stressful, they may panic or unexpectedly burst into tears. Pushing them too hard backfires with relapse and absence. Catching up has to be done *very* slowly. Extra praise and encouragement for the effort shown will be helpful.

There are several practical measures that need addressing too. Through no fault of their own, M.E. sufferers may need frequent visits to the loo; their food intolerances may involve bringing their own lunch and snacks. Low blood sugar may necessitate eating in class. Chemical sensitivities may make laboratory work difficult, although wearing a mask could help. These are available from Healthy House (see address at back of book).

Most of all, though, schoolchildren with M.E. need understanding and support. They are frequently embarrassed by their plight and will require sympathetic handling. A quiet word with the headteacher may be needed for this.

It is vital that you talk directly to your child's teacher about his or her needs. There is also an excellent booklet called *Guidelines for Schools*, written by Jane Colby, a former headmistress. When all teachers understand M.E., children will have a much better deal.

Parents need to make sure that travel arrangements are in hand and understand that homework and exams may have to be put on hold for the time being. It may even be necessary to take exams at home under supervision.

Sport and PE will not be possible for a while. Many people think that a bit of swimming is OK as the body is supported by the water. However, all the muscles are used and the vulnerable legs and knees work quite hard, and when I tried it a while ago my legs refused to move. This was quite a shock as I once held the senior breast-stroke record at my secondary school!

It may be unwise to enter into any immunisation programmes. Ask your doctor for advice on this.

Both parents and children will worry about loss of education. Children are quite intelligent enough to realise that eventually they will have to catch up, take exams and get a job, and this concerns them. Lots of reassurance and encouragement will be needed if they are not to give up.

Teenagers have special problems and needs during their growing-up years. With M.E., they lose out on experiences and friendships which shape and mould their lives for the future. Youngsters miss normal school life, their friends, social life, sport, musical activities, drama, walking the dog, hobbies, etc. Their lives are turned upside-down. They change from being overactive and full of energy to zombies, almost overnight sometimes. This leaves them frustrated, lonely, isolated, anxious, depressed and bored. It may take some time to accept this new 'geriatric' lifestyle and they may feel envious of their family and friends. Visits and letters from good, close friends could make all the difference during this trying time. This will keep them in touch with normality. The worst thing about M.E. is not knowing how long it is going to last. Relapses follow remissions, with natural disappointment, and your child's friends sometimes drop off one by one. Try to make sure your child is not forgotten.

Ordinary teenage problems are made worse by M.E. For example, how do you make and keep friends when you are hardly ever at school? If you muster up the energy to take a girl out one evening, how will you cope if *she* has to see *you* home, maybe carrying you? No, it is not funny! Try to help your child to adjust to these problems, to learn to look after himself really well, get better, then resume normal activity.

There will be some children who will not be able to attend school for quite lengthy periods of time (a year or more is quite common), and for these home tutoring will be a boon, if they are up to it. Just a few hours a week with a little bit of homework will help to keep things going. The sheer relief for parents and the reduced stress of the children who have been struggling at school can in itself bring about some immediate improvement. When the student feels ready to attempt a little bit of school again, it is essential to build the hours up slowly over a longish period.

Very young children

Fortunately, very few children of pre-school age seem to suffer from M.E., but it can happen. My specialist told me many years ago that he was treating new patients of two and 72. At both ends of this scale, M.E. will bring about very specific problems.

I have no personal experience of tiny children with M.E., but common sense suggests the situation would be much the same as with any other serious illness. However, the fluctuations of the illness would need to be taken into account on a daily basis. Whether ill or healthy, small children are very time-consuming and sick children would need amusing within their limitations of any particular day, which will vary considerably.

From a practical point of view, it could be quite difficult to leave a small child without someone really suitable being responsible, as the child may not be well enough some days to go out socially or even shopping in a pushchair on a cold day. Poorly children can be quite 'clingy' and need their mums and dads. They may not take kindly to 'aunties' or neighbours popping in for an hour.

Your biggest problem may be dealing with the child's exuberant energy on a good day, which will bring on a relapse the next day. Perhaps writing out a daily timetable together would help. This could incorporate short periods of active play, TV, tea in the garden, visits from friend, etc., alternating with quiet resting times.

You may be able to ease the situation by introducing a doll or teddy that is 'poorly' (with bandages, if necessary, to prove it!) and keeps the same routine as the sick child. Caring for the toy would help self-esteem and lessen boredom.

Some children may relate to a robot toy, or one they have seen on the television. When a robot or android breaks down, all you have to do is open a flap on the back and repair or replace the wiring system. You may be able to explain that our wiring system is more complicated and takes more time to mend itself slowly. We need extra rest for this to happen.

Keeping a bed-ridden child amused is difficult but not impossible. Puppets are a boon – finger puppets, glove puppets and even string puppets can be used. A very sleepy child can watch even if unable to participate. Plasticine and any kind of play dough are good for creativity. So are sticking things in scrap books, card games, noughts and crosses, magic painting and special pictures which you colour in one bit at a time, like painting by numbers. Maybe try keeping a weather chart, as they would at school, or making a birthday card. Children always love stories, whether in a recorded form, from story books or your own invention. Make their bedroom calm and relaxing but interesting too – mobiles and a musical box are good ideas.

When small children are really poorly, too ill to do anything much, but bored too, you may be able to make use of children's records played quietly or videos if they are up to it. Sometimes cuddling a small pet (a hamster or guinea pig) or watching a budgie or some goldfish may relieve the boredom and add interest to the day.

If going to the park is out of the question, try to make sure your child gets some fresh air on a warm day, even if it is only half an hour in the garden under a parasol. This will not only be healthy but provide a change of scenery from the lounge walls.

It is very sad to see such young children suffering in this way, but with good care and attention they stand the best chance of a full recovery. You may feel very helpless and inadequate at times, especially after a poor night's sleep, but just being there to support the child and giving out lots of love and security is all you can humanly be expected to do.

Carers

Carers will mostly be parents, who suddenly find themselves in a new, difficult situation for which nothing has prepared them. They have no experience to draw on, little knowledge of the illness and don't know how to handle it.

The first problem is acceptance, both by the parents and the child. Once everyone realises that the lifestyle of both the sufferer and, to some extent, that of the family will change, then you can get on with the job of collecting the information you will need, managing the illness appropriately and seeking further personal support.

As you may imagine, the main brunt of the extra work falls on the main carer, usually the mother. Her workload increases and she has to juggle time between a sick child's needs whilst trying hard not to neglect the needs of the other members of the family. Brothers and sisters may not understand at first and may feel quite confused. Families don't always understand the need for peace and quiet and the trials of sleep reversal. It can be very frustrating if you have finally fallen asleep after an awful night just as your brother starts his violin practice!

It is only natural for fit and healthy children to rush in and out of the house with friends, slamming doors and letting off steam after school, but this can be hell for the sufferer. Brothers and sisters sometimes may not even accept that the illness exists. Perhaps they are really worried about the long-term consequences should it prove to be true and maybe they fear they will catch it too.

Having a very poorly child in the house can affect plans for holidays, outings, food arrangements and general house rules. Yes, it does affect the *whole* family very much.

Very ill children may be depressed and emotional. They may shed extra tears or suddenly fly off the handle. They appear boring and unsociable. The rest of the family need to understand that this is part and parcel of the illness and learn to take it in their stride. Remember that emotional stress will cause huge setbacks for the illness, so try to diffuse tricky situations before they get out of hand.

Parents of M.E. sufferers may be worried about spoiling their children. It must be difficult to find a balance between caring and letting them get away with murder! Most parents use their instincts wisely, and the best advice I can give is to listen to the child and believe what is said. In times of frustration and disappointment, when things are going badly, some mums and dads may wonder what they are doing wrong. Feelings of guilt and inadequacy are natural but usually unnecessary. Certainly the parents I know are doing a great job, learning a new, impossible task for which they haven't been trained.

171

They combine housekeeper, nurse, counsellor, peacemaker and friend, usually in a few months. I am also amazed how quickly they become M.E. experts when the need arises. One mum explained to me that she just aims to hold everything together and keep some semblance of normality going, which just about sums it up. Carers everywhere, I take my hat off to you, the unsung heroes!

Last, but not least, I would point out that if a carer is to keep going and be of continuing use to the family, he/she will need a bit of space and personal quality time. With the best will in the world, it is not possible to spend every minute of the day worrying about M.E. and it would be counter-productive to do so. Carers have lives too and doing something quite different, enjoying a little outing or treat, will be necessary and good for you. So don't forget to look after yourself too!

CHAPTER 10

Conclusion

By now, you will realise what a serious, complicated illness M.E. is. I think of the recovery process as walking a tightrope at the top of a cliff: it is easy to fall off and it takes a long time to climb back up again! You may try some of my suggestions and feel like giving up as you do not notice any immediate or lasting benefit. Don't give up. Building up your immune system is a long job and an invisible one too. Perhaps, unknown to you, something has improved inside you, but it is just not enough yet to show any real difference. There may always be something just around the corner that will really help you. You will need a lot of patience and support, but hang in there.

Look at it this way: suppose you had a large hole in the garden which was originally going to be a lily pond. You now want to fill it in and make it into a patio. There is an enormous pile of gravel and earth for the job, but no spade – only a teaspoon! You are too tired to shovel more than half a dozen spoons a day but even though you seem to making no progress at all, eventually that hole will be filled! We are all dealing with that big, black hole, called M.E.

M.E. is an illness of remissions and relapses, and the relapses seem to predominate. It is so disappointing when you just start to improve, only to relapse again, perhaps due to an infection, overdoing it, stress or sometimes for no apparent reason at all. There is only one thing to do: 'Get back on your horse'. The statistics that do make sense are the ones that indicate that the majority of sufferers who take positive steps to help themselves do slowly improve.

For me, the key factors to improvement are rest, diet, supplements, relaxation, freedom from stress (including peace and quiet!) and a positive mental attitude. Above all, don't ever give up hope. I wish you good luck and good health.

Books, Audio Cassettes and Other Sources of Information

As well as books, there are many good factsheets and leaflets available from Action for M.E. (see page 179). These cover topics such as doctors, carers, education and patients' rights and there are separate sheets on such items as diet, magnesium injections, allergies, vitamins and candida. They also produce an introductory Therapy Information Pack (cost £3) and a video tape about M.E., and can provide a list of local support groups throughout the country.

You can also ring a 24-hour telephone information line which explains the causes and symptoms of M.E. and provides advice on diagnosis and lifestyle, finding sympathetic doctors and much more. Telephone Dr Anne Macintyre on 0891 122976. Calls are charged at 45p per minute cheap rate and 50p per minute at all other times, with 30 per cent of the revenue going to Action for M.E. funds.

If you join Action for M.E. or the M.E. Association you will automatically receive a number of useful information leaflets and their excellent journals.

Audio cassettes are very useful, especially if you are too ill to read. Action for M.E. produces tapes on items from their journal and relaxation tapes are a boon – see address list for suppliers.

Many health shops have a stock of leaflets, books and audio cassettes and your local library will order specialist books if you find them too expensive to buy. Below is a list of those I have found most useful.

Postviral Fatigue Syndrome, Leon Chaitow, J.M. Dent & Sons Ltd.

M.E. Post-Viral Fatigue Syndrome: How to Live With It, Dr Anne Macintyre, Thorsons.

Living with M.E., Dr Charles Shepherd, Cedar.

Fibromyalgia and Muscle Pain, Leon Chaitow. Thorsons.

Arthritis – The Allergy Connection, Dr John Mansfield, Thorsons.

Food Allergy and Intolerance, Dr Jonathan Brostoff and Linda Gamlin, Bloomsbury.

Food Combining Diet, Kathryn Marsden, Thorsons.

Stress – How Your Diet Can Help, Stephen Terrass, Thorsons.

Low Blood Sugar, Martin and Maggie Budd, Thorsons.

Candida Albicans, Leon Chaitow, Thorsons.

Candida Albicans Yeast-free Recipes for Renewed Health and Vitality, Richard Turner and Elizabeth Simonsen, Thorsons.

The Liver Cleansing Diet, Dr Sandra Cabot

Evening Primrose Oil, Judy Graham, Thorsons.

Today's Herbal Health, Louise Tenney, Woodland Books, PO Box 160, Pleasant Grove, UT 84062, USA. Probably available in health shops.

Garlic for Health, David Roser, Martin Books.

Barefoot Homoeopath, Madeleine Harland and Glen Finn, Hyden House Ltd.

Reflexology, Nicola M. Hall, Thorsons.

Talking about Acupuncture, J. R. Worsley, Element Books.

The Holistic Approach to Detoxification and Colon Care, Anne Shulman, Green Library.

The Back and Beyond, Dr Paul Sherwood, Arrowbooks.

Thyroid Problems, Patsy Wescott, Thorsons.

Are You Sleeping in a Safe Place?, Rolf Gordon, self-published.

Children with M.E., Dr Alan Franklin FRCP, DCH, Action for M.E.

Guidelines for Schools, Jane Colby, Action for M.E.

Useful Addresses

Action Groups

Action for M.E.
PO Box 1302, Wells, Somerset, BA5 2WE.
Office hours 9 am – 5 pm, Monday to Friday.
Tel: 01749 670799 (Non-members)
01749 670577 (Members)
01749 670402 (Counselling)
01749 330105 (Benefits Helpline)
01227 263454 (Therapy Information Line)
01992 632616 (Welfare Benefits Advice).

Action for M.E.'s journal *InterAction* (£4.50) is available from:
Zoe Williams
4 St. Denys Close, Stanford-in-the-Vale,
Faringdon, Oxon, SN7 8NJ.

The M.E. Association
Stanhope House, 4 Corringham Road,
Stanford-le-Hope, Essex, SS17 0HA.
Tel: 01375 642466 (Office hours: 9 am – 12.30 pm, 1.30 pm – 4.45 pm)
01375 361013 (Advice Line: 1.30 pm – 4 pm)
After 5 pm, ring 01375 642466 for numbers for that particular evening.

The Carers National Association
20–25 Glasshouse Yard, London, EC1A 4JS.
Tel: 0171 490 8818

The National M.E. Centre
Harold Wood Hospital, Gubbins Lane,
Harold Wood, Romford, Essex, RM3 0BE.
Tel: 01708 378050

Action against Allergy
24–26 High Street, Hampton Hill, Middlesex,
TW12 1PD.

**The Fund for Osteopathic Research into M.E.
(FORME)**
83 Whittaker Lane, Prestwich, Manchester, M25
1ET. (Charity number 1045005).

Osteopathic Information Service
Box 2074, Reading, Berkshire, RG1 4YR
Tel: 0118 951 2051

Professional Associations

The National Institute of Medical Herbalists
9 Palace Gate, Exeter, Devon, EX1 1JA.
Tel: 01392 426022

The Royal Homoeopathic Hospital
(This is a National Health Hospital)
60 Great Ormond Street, London, WC1N 3HR.
Tel: 0171 837 8833

The Society of Homoeopaths
2 Artizan Road, Northampton, NN1 4HU.
Tel: 01604 21400

The Association for Systemic Kinesiology
39 Browns Road, Surbiton, Surrey, KT5 8ST.
Tel: 0181 399 3215

The British Massage Therapy Council
9 Elm Road, Worthing, W. Sussex, BN11 1PG.
Tel: 01293 775467

The Chartered Society of Physiotherapy (CSP)
14 Bedford Road, London, WC1R 4ED.
Tel: 0171 242 1941

The Council for Acupuncture
179 Gloucester Road, London, NW1 6DX.
Tel: 0171 724 5756

**The Acupuncture Association of Chartered
Physiotherapists (AACP)**
Holly House, 6 Barncroft Road,
Berkhamsted, Herts, HP4 3NL.
Tel: 01442 864243

**The Organisation of Chartered Physiotherapists
in Private Practice (OCPPP)**
855A London Road, Westcliff on Sea,
Essex, SS0 9SZ.
Tel: 01702 77462

The Association of Reflexologists
27 Old Gloucester Street, London, WC1 3XX.
Tel: 01273 479020

The British Thyroid Foundation
PO Box HP22, Leeds, LS6 3RT.

The British Tinnitus Association
14–18 West Bar Green, Sheffield, S1 2DA.

Suppliers

The Healthy House
(for equipment for allergy-prone people, e g. dust-mite-proof bedding)
Cold Harbour, Ruscombe, Stroud,
Glos., GL6 6DA.
Tel: 01453 752216

BioCare Ltd
(for supplements)
54 Northfield Road, Kings Norton,
Birmingham B30 1JH.
Tel: 0121 433 3727

Biolab
(for tests – doctor's letter required).
The Stone House, 9 Weymouth Street,
London W1N 3FF.
Tel: 0171 636 5959

Blackmores Laboratories Ltd
(for information only)
Unit 7, Poyle Tech Centre, Willow Road, Poyle,
Colnbrook, Bucks.

The Green Library
(for books on health matters)
Homewood NHS Trust (DHQ), Guildford Road,
Chertsey, Surrey, KT16 0QA.
Tel: 01932 874333

Dulwich Health
130 Gipsy Hill, London, SE19 1PL.
Tel: 0181 670 5883

Lamberts Healthcare Ltd
(for supplements)
1 Lamberts Road, Tunbridge Wells,
Kent, TN2 3EQ.
Tel: 01892 552119

Larkhall
(for supplements)
Green Farm, 225 Putney Bridge Road,
London, SW15 2BR.
Tel: 0181 874 1130 or 0181 874 5631

Full Spectrum Lighting Limited
(for light boxes)
Unit 1, Riverside Business Centre, Victoria Street,
High Wycombe, Buckinghamshire, HP11 2LT.
Tel: 01494 526051

The Real Meat Co. Ltd
(for organic meat)
East Hill Farm, Heytesbury, Warminster,
Wiltshire, BA12 0HR.
Tel: 01985 40436

Swaddles Green Farm
Hare Lane, Buckland St. Mary, Chard, Somerset,
TA20 3JR.
24hr answerphone for orders: 01460 234387

New World Aurora
(for relaxation tapes)
New World Cassettes, 16A Neal's Yard,
Covent Garden, London WC2.
Tel: 0171 379 5972

Mail order address:
New World Cassettes, Paradise Farm, Westhall,
Halesworth, Suffolk, IP19 8RH.
Tel: 0198 681682

Simply Sausages
(open Mon. to Fri. 8 am – 6 pm, Sat. 9 am – 2 pm)
Harts Corner, 341 Central Markets,
Farringdon Street, London, EC1A 9BN.
Tel: 0171 329 3227

Solgar Vitamins Ltd
(for information only)
Solgar House, New Ground Farm,
New Ground Road, Aldbury, Herts.
Tel: 01442 890355

G & G Supplies
(for Superdophilus)
175 London Road, East Grinstead, Sussex.

Claire Monk
(for VEGA testing and electro-acupuncture)
50 Bodmin Road, Luton, Beds.
Tel: 01582 579148

Author's Note on Roger Rose

Mr Roger Rose died suddenly in the summer of 1997, shortly after I finished the manuscript for this book.

Over the years, this unique gentleman brought help and comfort to many thousands of people, including myself, through not only his expertise and experience, but also his friendly manner and gentle sense of humour.

I, and many other M.E. sufferers, regarded him as a our safety net and felt secure in the knowledge that he could diagnose and provide treatment for all those miserable conditions which exacerbated our M.E. from time to time. He was a delightful man who always took the time to explain everything beautifully, put other people's needs before financial gain and earned respect from everyone who knew him. He was wholly absorbed by his work and continued to see patients when well past retirement age.

He was a good friend who will be missed by so many people. However, his work will not die with him, thanks to his protegée, Claire Monk, who will continue his practice. I hope that this book will be seen as a fitting tribute to him.

Index

187